Knowledge Is Power

What Every Woman Should Know
about Breast Cancer

Dr. Dennis L. Citrin

Edited by Catherine D. Driscoll

ISBN-13: 9781493573561

ISBN-10: 149357356X

Library of Congress Control Number: 2013920489
CreateSpace Independent Publishing Platform
North Charleston, South Carolina

Knowledge Is Power

What Every Woman Should Know about Breast Cancer

By Dr. Dennis L. Citrin

Edited by Catherine D. Driscoll

Foreword

There are likely few adult members of our society who have not in some manner been touched by the diagnosis of breast cancer, whether as a result of their own diagnosis, or that of a spouse, family member, or close friend.

First, there is the anxiety of waiting for results of a screening mammogram or a subsequent evaluation because something abnormal was suspected.

Then there is the impact of therapy itself: the effects of breast surgery, radiation, and chemotherapy on one's body image; the psychological well-being of the patient; concerns with both short-term and longer-term side effects; and questions about the ability to carry on with one's daily life during and following treatment.

And finally, there are the questions that lurk in the shadows: "Am I cured?" "Will the cancer recur?" "How long will I live?" "What will happen next and when?" "What can I do myself to improve the chances that the cancer will not recur or that my survival will be as long as possible?"

The medical condition known as "breast cancer" actually represents many different forms of the disease with varying recommended treatments. These treatments are based on a large number of factors, including features of the tumor itself (stage, the presence or absence of particular biological markers) and features specific to the individual patient (a history of heart disease or other preexisting medical conditions).

It is with this background of widespread uncertainty and concern by so many that we welcome this excellent new book written by Dr. Dennis Citrin, a nationally recognized medical oncologist and expert in the management of breast cancer. Based on his forty years of experience, Dr. Citrin has written a book for patients, families, friends, and all nonmedical members of society to address our critically important questions and concerns. Dr. Citrin's book breaks down the facts about breast cancer and helps explain this very complex disease, its management, and perhaps most importantly, what patients can do themselves to ensure the best possible outcomes.

What makes this book unique and even more powerful are the commentaries provided by Dr. Citrin's own patients. Representing different ages, ethnicities, and cultures, these brave women share their personal stories of how they dealt with their diagnosis, treatment and side effects, their uncertainties, and their futures. The messages conveyed in the words on these pages are insightful and inspiring and provide a powerful message of hope for all women.

Maurie Markman, MD

Senior Vice President of Clinical Affairs & National Director of Medical Oncology
Cancer Treatment Centers of America

Table of Contents

Introduction

"I have a zest for life today. I want to teach people, to tell people what I've been through, so that other women don't make the same mistakes."
—*Sandra Dillahunty*

Every week, approximately 4,000 women are diagnosed with breast cancer in the United States. Despite this considerable impact on more than two hundred thousand women every year, the timely diagnosis and appropriate treatment of breast cancer remains less than perfect.

Two recent studies I conducted showed that in 16 percent of patients with breast cancer (nearly one in six patients), there was a delay of at least six months in obtaining a cancer diagnosis or starting treatment. In the second study, a large number of patients failed to follow the treatment recommendations of their care specialists (oncologists). One half of all patients who were prescribed estrogen-blocking drugs (endocrine treatment) did not complete the treatment plans suggested by their doctors.

As a medical oncologist who has spent nearly forty years dedicated to helping women survive breast cancer, I struggle to understand what drives those statistics when public awareness and our understanding of the disease is so high and treatment is so effective.

Every year I treat hundreds of women, many who continue to thrive and live happily for many years after they have been diagnosed with breast cancer. My job is to educate them, help them understand what is happening, and give them treatment choices they can accept and follow. I find that when patients are fully educated and invited to become a partner in developing their treatment plans, they can overcome their fears and act quickly to make more educated decisions.

Most breast cancers are highly curable, but every breast cancer is potentially fatal. If you remember only three things after reading this book, I hope they are:

- **Don't delay getting a diagnosis.** Breast cancer is a highly treatable disease, and most patients diagnosed with early stage disease can confidently expect to be totally cured. So if you feel a lump in your breast, see your doctor immediately. It will not go away on its own.
- **Follow your treatment plan.** Breast cancer is a chronic illness; as such, treatment often extends over years. It is critically important that patients with breast cancer understand this and are able to completely commit to extended treatment and observation to prevent the cancer from recurring.
- **If you suspect or know you have cancer, seek professional medical advice and opinions from reputable sources.** Cancer cannot be cured with chiropractics or yoga or vitamins or diet. Holistic and naturopathic approaches are very beneficial for women to reduce the side effects of cancer treatment, but those approaches will not *by themselves* cure cancer. An integrative approach that includes medical treatment and holistic therapies is best.

Many of my patients at CTCA at Midwestern Regional Medical Center (Midwestern) have graciously shared their stories in this book. I hope you learn from them. These women are living, breathing examples of the power of prompt diagnosis and effective treatment, and they share their stories here to help others.

* * *

Over the past thirty years or so, we have learned a great deal about breast cancer. Many innovations in cancer medicine have made earlier diagnosis of breast cancer possible and treatment more effective and tolerable. So today, breast cancer is a highly treatable disease, and most patients with early stage breast cancer can confidently expect to be totally cured.

Every breast patient with cancer is unique, just as each cancer is unique. There is a wide spectrum of breast cancers that range from very slow-growing cancers, which are easily treated and pose little threat to the patient's life if properly treated, to highly malignant, very aggressive, and fast-growing cancers, in which accurate diagnosis and prompt treatment are essential if the patient's life is to be saved. As such, treatment plans are as individual as the patient and her cancer.

It is very natural for a woman diagnosed with breast cancer to experience real fear. But no woman can let fear delay diagnosis or seeking appropriate treatment. Breast cancer is a treatable disease if diagnosed early and treated thoroughly. It's important to seek medical advice as soon as possible to ensure the best possible outcome. Patients must overcome their fears to take advantage of the science that is available.

The medical community continues to learn about breast cancer, and every patient who has the disease deserves access to that knowledge. Patients should expect their medical teams to fully explain everything about their cancer, diagnosis, and treatment options. If you don't understand something, ask questions. The more educated a patient is, the more likely she will be able to overcome fear and anxiety and to make the best treatment decisions for herself. Your life is really in your hands, so you must learn to be your own advocate.

And last, I firmly believe that the best treatment results come when patients have access to a dedicated breast cancer treatment team comprised of surgical and medical oncologists, pathologists, radiologists, nutritionists, naturopathic providers, and mind-body therapists. In addition to educating and treating the patient, a team approach ensures that the patient has the medical, spiritual, and emotional support she needs to fight and win her battle against breast cancer.

In this book, we will describe what every woman facing breast cancer should know about the disease. You will learn about the importance of early diagnosis and why you should choose a physician or treatment team that provides good physician/patient communication. Good communication is essential to ensuring a prompt diagnosis and correct treatment decisions. We will discuss the numerous treatment options that are now available for the patient diagnosed with breast cancer and describe what I believe to be the best breast cancer treatment approach available, the CTCA Integrative Breast Cancer Care Model. And last, we will describe unique clinical problems that require special consideration.

I strongly believe that a knowledgeable and informed patient is her own best advocate.

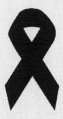

Denial is not a plan.

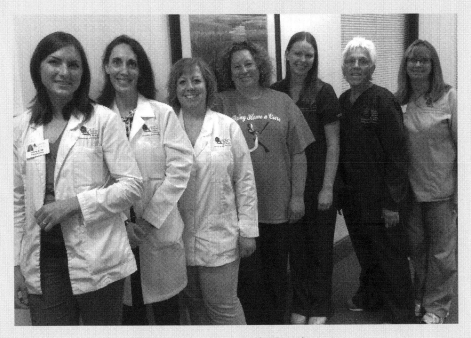

"I didn't have anything to fear.
I should have known better than to delay treatment."
—Jennifer Barber, *center, with members of her breast cancer team*

IN NOVEMBER 2010, JENNIFER BARBER, a young, vibrant mom from Kenosha, Wisconsin, felt a lump in her right breast. She knew something was wrong, but she didn't want to confront it.

"I did a lot of research online," Jennifer says, "and learned that most lumps are not cancerous but just cysts. I knew I should have it checked out. But I was fearful, so I let it go for six or seven months. It got larger and larger. I'm a stomach sleeper, and it began to be uncomfortable."

Then she found a lump under her arm and finally sought medical help in May 2011. By then, the cancer in her breast had increased significantly in size and had spread to the lymph nodes in her right armpit.

When I first examined Jennifer in June 2011, the right breast contained a very large mass, measuring ten centimeters in diameter (about five inches), with a large cancerous lymph node in the right armpit.

She was treated with chemotherapy from June until August 2011. Jennifer handled the treatment very well, and with chemotherapy, the large tumor masses in the breast and the lymph node disappeared almost completely.

"I had heard how horrible chemotherapy was and began to prepare myself for that rollercoaster," Jennifer says. "But it wasn't at all what I expected. After the first chemo, I felt a little nauseous. They gave me medication for it, and it went away within an hour. From then on, I felt fine and had no problems at all."

Throughout her treatment, Jennifer vowed to eat healthier foods to help her body fight her cancer. "Everyone has vices—smoking, drinking, whatever. Mine was poor nutrition. As a busy mom with kids, it was easier to swing in a drive-through than to fix something healthy. But I've turned that around now. I've learned from the registered dietician that I need to feed my body so that I can fight this cancer. No more drive-throughs for me!"

By the time Jennifer came to surgery in September 2011, there was no sign of any residual cancer in her breast and lymph nodes. All of the tissue my surgical colleague removed was simply scar tissue left from the destroyed cancer cells.

Jennifer needed several more chemotherapy treatments and then radiation to the breast and armpit. Her prognosis for a complete cure is excellent.

"My experience was the opposite of what I was expecting," Jennifer says. "I've gotten back to my life so quickly. In fact, cancer hasn't interrupted my life or my family's life at all. It's just been a little bump in the road. Fear played a big role in my not wanting to get checked out. But I didn't have anything to fear. I should have known better. If I had confronted it six months earlier, it could have been much better."

Jennifer's advice to others: no matter how small, get it checked out. "Chemo treatment is not a big deal. There are great meds for the side effects now. It has been a wonderful, positive experience for me. I feel so good about being in the right place."

Doctor's Comments

It is very natural to be frightened if you feel a lump in your breast, but you mustn't allow that fear to stop you from seeking immediate medical help.

Jennifer waited six months before seeking medical help, and during those six months, the very aggressive and fast-growing cancer more than doubled in size. Thankfully, she responded very well to chemotherapy treatment. As a result, she did not have to lose her breast, and her prognosis for total cure is excellent.

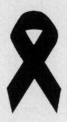

Trust Your Instincts.

CYNTHIA OLMSTEAD WAS MINUTES AWAY from having her right breast removed when her neighbor delivered her mail. In it was a letter that said, "We have interpreted your radiology examination and are pleased to report that it shows no evidence of breast cancer." It was the same letter she'd received in 2008 after a mammogram, three ultrasounds, an MRI with dye, a stereotactic biopsy, and a lumpectomy that showed "benign" breast tissue in the sample.

Cynthia was fifty-eight years old in March 2008 when she complained of pain in her left breast. While a mammogram showed no abnormality in the *left* breast where she had pain, it did show a suspicious area in the *right* breast.

After an ultrasound and MRI examination of the right breast, Cynthia had a needle biopsy in April 2008. The biopsy was negative for cancer, but her surgeon was so suspicious that she recommended surgical removal of the area. The surgery was done in May 2008, and once again it was reported as benign tissue with no evidence of cancer.

Cynthia was concerned because she felt a lump after surgery but was told that this was simply bruising from the surgery. When she returned for her next mammogram in October 2009, she showed the area to the technologist and requested an ultrasound examination, but the medical staff wouldn't order an ultrasound. Why? Because the mammogram she had in 2009 had been normal.

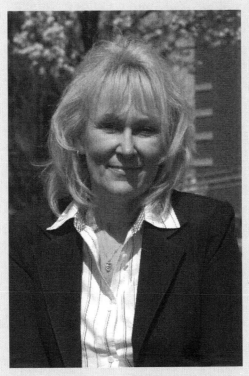

"I wish I'd known that never missing a single annual mammogram in twenty years was no guarantee that we'd catch any sign of breast cancer early."
—*Cynthia Olmstead*

"No one wants to look for trouble," Cynthia says, "and my doctor was absolutely sure that there was no cancer there."

In August 2010, Cynthia consulted her gynecologist because her right breast still felt very abnormal to her. Her gynecologist reassured her that everything was "fine" because her 2009 mammogram had been normal.

Cynthia was still concerned in October 2010. By then, the area was much larger, and her right nipple had started to invert. Her annual mammogram was once again reported as normal. Despite this, she insisted on seeing a surgeon, who immediately performed a biopsy, confirming the presence of invasive lobular carcinoma.

Cynthia had a mastectomy in November 2010. At that time, the tumor in the right breast measured five centimeters in size. She was started on adjuvant hormone treatment. When last seen in August 2013, she remains cancer free.

"I wish I'd known that never missing a single annual mammogram in twenty years was no guarantee that we'd catch any sign of breast cancer early—even though technicians saw and felt the lump in my breast," Cynthia shares. "I wish I'd sought a second opinion in 2009, when the mammography technician simply waved me out the door with a cheery, 'Everything's fine,' instead of ordering an immediate ultrasound on that lump. I wish I'd trusted my instincts sooner…but I so wanted to believe that coveted, pleased-to-report letter telling me there was 'no evidence of breast cancer' in my body that I didn't pay attention to instincts.

"Mammograms are NOT the end-all to breast cancer diagnosis. Just ask me. I know. I never missed one. Not one."

Doctor's Comments

Cynthia's story is very typical of patients with lobular carcinoma of the breast. In contrast to ductal carcinoma (which is much more common), lobular carcinoma is notoriously difficult to diagnose for two reasons: It often doesn't produce an obvious lump in the breast, but presents as a subtle area of thickening that many doctors find unimpressive. Second, it is frequently not visible on the mammogram.

It is important to emphasize that a negative mammogram IN NO WAY excludes breast cancer in any woman who complains of a persistent lump in her breast.

If you feel something wrong with your breast, don't allow yourself to be reassured that "everything's fine." You have to have the issue fully investigated. If you're not satisfied with what you're hearing from your doctor, seek a second opinion.

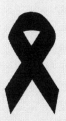

Alternative therapies can be helpful, but not by themselves a cure.

SANDRA DILLAHUNTY FIRST FELT A LUMP in her left breast in November 2003 when she was fifty-five years old. She was a strong believer in natural healing; she'd never been seriously ill in her life and had been raised to believe that the body can heal itself when given the right resources. "My father literally died overnight from polio, so my mother never had much faith in 'white coats.' We are not doctor people," she says.

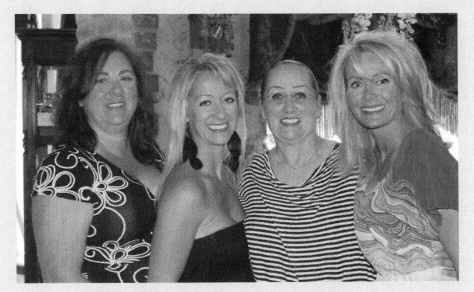

"The cancer is not ever going to go away on its own. It has to be removed. You can't look for an easy way out."
—Sandra Dillahunty, shown with her daughters

Sandra did see a doctor, however, who obtained a needle biopsy (tissue sample) from the left breast and confirmed the diagnosis of breast cancer.

The doctor recommended surgery, but Sandra declined all conventional cancer treatment. Instead, she chose to receive four years of alternative treatment from a doctor in Texas. His program involved regular injections of hydrogen peroxide, removal of all of her dental fillings (which he told her were the cause of her cancer), colon cleanses, shock treatments delivered through a waistband, wearing a hat designed to remove parasites from her body that she was told could be causing the cancer, and juicing.

During the four years she endured this alternative treatment, her weight fell to ninety-eight pounds, and she could feel her tumor continuing to grow. She spent more than two hundred thousand dollars on these "treatments."

By the time Sandra came to CTCA in October 2007, she had a very advanced cancer that occupied most of her left breast. The disease had also spread to her liver and lungs. Sandra required a mastectomy followed by oral chemotherapy. She remained in remission on this treatment for nearly three years. In 2011, she developed multiple skin nodules in her left mastectomy scar. She started on an oral Aromatase Inhibitor (hormone therapy), and the skin nodules rapidly resolved.

More recently Sandra started intraveneous chemotherapy to control a chest wall recurrence of her disease. Overall, she feels well and is fully active.

Since starting her treatment at CTCA, Sandra's attitude about medical care has completely changed. "It's not a death sentence. It's just cancer," she says. "If you were diagnosed with diabetes, you'd be treated for it. So you can't look for an easy way out because it won't go away. Surgery is no fun, believe me, but it was necessary. And the other treatments I endured were much worse and not effective. The cancer is not ever going to go away on its own. It has to be removed."

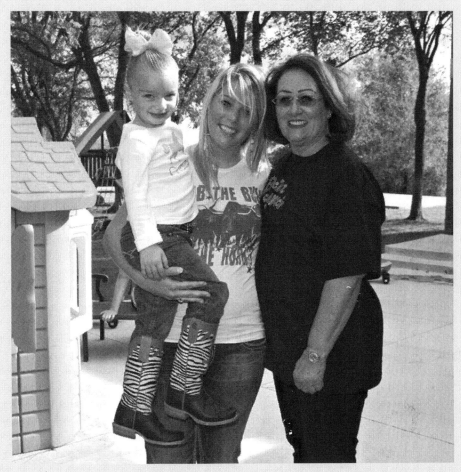

Sandra Dillahunty (right) with her daughter and granddaughter

As for chemotherapy, Sandra says, "Chemo won't kill you. It's just a drug, like any other drug. You'll get through it. I hear women say that they're afraid of losing their hair. It's just hair! We shave it off of our legs every day! Go get a wig—it is not a big deal.

"I have a zest for life today," Sandra says. "I want to teach people, to tell people what I've been through so that other women don't make the same mistakes. I give glory to God for healing me...body, soul, and mind."

Doctor's Comments

Many women who are diagnosed with breast cancer refuse some or all of the treatment recommended by their doctors. Instead they try to control their disease with wholly unproven "cancer treatments" that they often learn about through the Internet.

Sandra endured nearly four years of painful and expensive alternative therapies that did not control her breast cancer. She has been receiving treatment at CTCA for six years and continues to lead an active lifestyle.

CHAPTER 1

What Is Breast Cancer?

"Cancer was never a chapter that I wanted in my book.
But I wouldn't trade all I've learned because of this experience.
To laugh, to connect with beautiful people, to appreciate my life.
That's what I've learned."
— Andrea Gildner

How Cancer Cells Grow and Invade

The human body is composed of billions of microscopic cells. Normally these cells live and function in perfect harmony with their neighbors. But sometimes they don't.

An important characteristic of living tissues and organs is their ability to grow. Growth of living tissue occurs through the process of cell division, where one cell becomes two cells, two cells become four cells, and so on.

Cell growth and division are an essential aspect of our lives. It's through cell growth that the body repairs itself from disease or injury. For example, when you cut your hand, the skin cells immediately begin to divide to make new skin cells to heal the cut. Such cell growth is tightly controlled. As soon as the cut in your hand is healed, the increased cell growth ceases.

In cancer cells, for reasons that are often not fully understood, the normal control mechanisms that govern cell division don't function properly. Instead of *controlled* cell growth, there is *uncontrolled* growth of abnormal cells, which leads to the development of a mass of abnormal cells, forming a lump or tumor.

Worse, the highly abnormal cells that form a cancerous tumor have the ability to destroy normal healthy cells and to travel from their original location to invade other tissues. Normally skin cells stay in the skin, lung cells stay in the lung, breast cells remain in the breast, and so on. But cancer cells that originate in these tissues don't respect normal tissue boundaries and have the ability to invade other organs, either by direct spread, through blood vessels, or through tiny channels *(lymphatic vessels)* that transport tissue fluid.

When cancer cells spread throughout the body, they eventually cause serious damage to vital organs, such as the lung, liver, or brain. And that is what ultimately kills the patient.

How and Why Breast Cancer Forms

Most breast cancers originate from the cells that line the milk ducts in the breast. Although almost every cell in the human body can become cancerous, most human cancers originate in cells that form the lining tissue of organs. We call these cancers *carcinomas*, and almost all of the common cancers that we deal with (cancers of the breast, bowel, stomach, lung, pancreas, bladder, cervix, uterus, ovary, and skin) are carcinomas.

Exactly why the lining cells of the breast ducts become cancerous is not known. It is generally true that when tissue is damaged over many years and cells are stimulated to grow in response to that damage, cancerous changes in the cells are more likely to occur. (Think of skin cells damaged by repeated exposure to ultraviolet radiation from the sun or the cells that line the major airways in the lung damaged for years by the chemicals in tobacco smoke.)

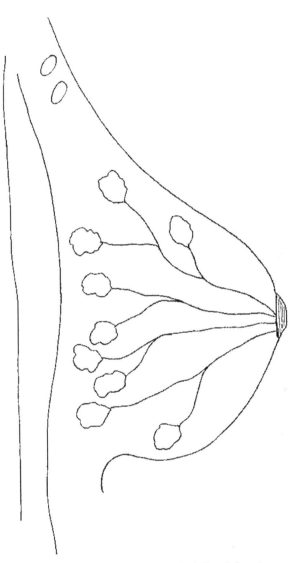

The normal breast is composed of glandular tissue
(lobules and ducts). Interspersed between the breast tissue is fat.

In the case of breast cancer, there isn't such an easily recognized factor that causes tissue damage. But we do know that the cells that line the milk ducts are very sensitive to stimulation by female sex hormones, particularly estrogen. Estrogen stimulates breast cells to divide and grow. Estrogen causes young girls' breasts to grow when they go through puberty and causes most women to experience some pain, heaviness, or tenderness in their breasts just before their periods.

The effect of estrogen on cell growth explains why taking additional estrogen (either as postmenopausal hormone replacement, or in the now-obsolete, high-dose estrogen oral contraceptive pills popular during the 1950s and 1960s) increases a woman's risk for developing breast cancer.

The stimulation caused by estrogen also explains why men have such a tiny risk for developing breast cancer. Men have all the same equipment in their breasts that women have—breast ducts and milk glands, albeit in a very undeveloped form. But in men, these cells are not being stimulated on a monthly basis by estrogen.

Many years ago, men were treated for prostate cancer with estrogen. As a side effect of this treatment, their breasts would swell and become tender (doctors call this condition *gynecomastia*). So doctors gave radiation to the breasts to prevent gynecomastia from developing. The combination of low-dose radiation and estrogen actually caused these men to develop breast cancer.

What causes breast cancer in women?

Estrogen produced naturally by the woman's ovaries or taken as medication stimulates the cells that line the ducts of the breast to grow, and whenever there is an increase in cell growth, there is a chance for abnormal cell growth, leading to precancerous cells and ultimately to cancer.

For reasons that are not clear, the ductal cells of some women are more likely to develop precancerous tissue damage than others. But it is difficult to identify these women. Some have a family history of breast cancer. Others have a specific gene mutation (*BRCA* or Breast Cancer Gene) that can be identified through a blood test.

But every woman should consider herself at some risk for developing breast cancer. It is critically important for all women to educate themselves about breast cancer and receive routine screenings or mammograms to detect the disease.

Stages of Breast Cancer Development

Breast cancer cells originate in the tissue that lines the tiny milk ducts in the breasts. The growth of those cells progresses through several phases until invasive cancer develops. This process can take years. The good news is that these abnormal cells can often be identified through a screening mammogram (breast X-ray) long before true invasive cancer is present. Preinvasive cancer, also known as *Ductal Carcinoma in Situ* (DCIS), is usually recognized on the mammogram by the presence of microscopic areas of calcification.

According to the American Cancer Society, there were 57,650 new cases of DCIS in 2011, the most recent year for which statistics are available. So that means that more than fifty thousand women per year *do not* develop invasive breast cancer because they practice excellent preventive medicine by having yearly screening mammograms.

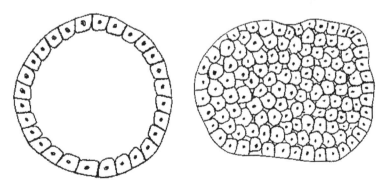

Above left: Cross section of a normal duct showing a single layer of normal ductal cells.
Above right: Cross section showing an increase in the number of normal appearing cells (ductal hyperplasia).

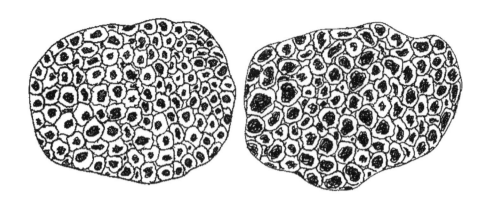

Above left: Duct is completely filled; cells are bigger than normal, darker than normal. Atypical ductal hyperplasia. Increase in number of cells that appear abnormal (or atypical).

Above right: Ductal Carcinoma in Situ (DCIS)
The duct is filled with very abnormal-appearing cells that are large, irregular, and dark-staining, as they contain abnormal DNA. These are cancer cells that have not yet progressed outside of the duct.

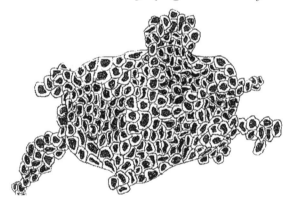

Above: Invasive Ductal Carcinoma with Residual DCIS. The abnormal appearing cancer cells have now spread beyond the confines of the duct and invaded into the surrounding fatty tissue of the breast.

DCIS is easily treated (never with chemotherapy) and almost 100 percent curable. Patients with DCIS are living, breathing advertisements for the value of regular screening mammograms.

If DCIS is not identified and promptly treated, abnormal breast cancer cells begin growing through the walls of the milk ducts and invade the surrounding fatty tissue of the breast. This is *invasive carcinoma*. Continued growth of these cancer cells will ultimately result in the formation of a mass, lump, or tumor (the names are interchangeable).

Most cases of invasive breast cancer are still completely curable as long as the patient is treated appropriately. Problems arise, however, when the disease is not diagnosed before it spreads to distant areas or proper treatment is not employed. Breast cancer cells that are not recognized and destroyed will continue to form new cancer cells and will eventually spread to other parts of the body. Untreated, the tumor will increase in size and will eventually spread to surrounding structures, typically the skin of the breast and the muscles of the chest wall.

Untreated for many months, breast cancer will eventually destroy the skin of the breast, producing large ulcerated masses that can bleed or become infected and cause the patient pain and severe discomfort. The cancerous tumor can also directly attach to the chest wall where it becomes fixed to the muscles, ribs, or breastbone and cannot be easily removed. Fortunately, such cases of locally advanced breast cancer are relatively rare today, except in cases when the patient has either delayed seeking medical help or refused conventional treatment.

Breast cancer cells can also spread through the lymphatic system or the blood stream, developing secondary tumors known as *metastases* in areas of the body distant from the breast. The first place for metastases to develop is in the lymph nodes of the armpit (axilla).

The importance of these nodes is twofold. First, if cancer is present in one or more nodes, the nodes must be surgically removed and are usually treated with radiation. Second and just as important, if cancer has already spread into the axillary lymph nodes at the time of first diagnosis, it is likely that cancer cells may have also spread to more distant areas of the body.

Here is an analogy to explain why this is so important: Imagine you're sitting in a big movie theater, and the movie has just finished. You wait for a minute before you stand up to leave and see people standing in the exits. Since you waited to stand and leave, it is likely the people in front of you are not the *first* people to leave the theater—others have probably already left before them.

Likewise, if there are cancer cells present in the axillary nodes under the armpits (detected during surgery), then there is a high probability that some cancer cells have already left the "theater" and are heading elsewhere in the body. These are the cancer cells that are likely to cause trouble years later unless they are destroyed through drug treatment.

So it is very important to determine at the time of first diagnosis whether there are identifiable cancer cells in the axillary lymph nodes. Knowing this provides crucial information to you and your doctor regarding your prognosis (the probability of cure versus relapse) and is critical to developing an effective treatment plan.

What kills the patient with breast cancer?

Some types of cancer are fatal to the patient because of where the cancer is *located* and how it interferes with the function of an essential organ. For example, cancer in the brain causes a fatal rise in pressure within the skull, or a brain hemorrhage. Cancer in the lung causes severe pneumonia and lung failure. Cancer in the bowel causes bowel obstruction.

How does breast cancer kill patients? The simple answer is that in some patients, the cancer spreads to distant parts of the body before the primary cancer in the breast has been identified or removed. We call this phenomenon *occult metastatic disease* because these cells that have spread are initially undetectable. We can't see them in CAT scans or MRIs, detect them through sophisticated blood tests, or identify their presence in distant sites at the time the cancer is first diagnosed. But we know that they are there because eventually the cells that "left the theater" will grow to a size and number that will eventually cause enough symptoms to the patient to be detected. But it is often many years after the primary tumor in the breast is recognized and treated.

And that is when we say that the cancer has *recurred,* or the patient has *relapsed.*

Every year, thousands of women experience a relapse of their disease in bone, liver, skin, or other distant sites, years after being treated successfully with local treatment (surgery and radiation) to destroy the cancer in the breast and lymph nodes in the axilla (armpit). It is possible for a relapse to occur at a distant site without experiencing a relapse on the chest wall where the cancerous breast (or part of the breast) was removed.

Recurrent breast cancer can take many forms. In approximately 50 percent of relapsing patients, the first area of recurrence is in the chest wall or axilla (armpit), near where the original cancer was located. Doctors call this *loco-regional recurrence.* In other patients, the first recurrence occurs at a distant site (bone, liver, or lung).

Determining a Prognosis

A good prognosis means a low probability of future recurrence of cancer with a high probability of complete cure. A poor prognosis indicates a high probability of future recurrence of the disease, resulting in death from breast cancer.

Prognostic factors are the medical facts that help a cancer doctor more accurately predict what the prognosis is for any individual patient. Negative prognostic factors increase the risk of relapse, while positive factors increase the probability of cure.

None of us has a crystal ball; we cannot predict with 100 percent certainty. But we do know a great deal about the relevant factors that make one breast cancer potentially more lethal than another.

Prognostic factors are divided into two major groups: those that relate to the stage of disease, and those that reflect the biologic nature of the tumor. Doctors refer to these factors as *staging* and *biology*, which will be discussed later.

What are the signs of breast cancer?

Breast cancer is a very treatable and curable disease, as long as it is diagnosed early and treated properly. That's why women must **pay attention to their bodies**, be their own best advocates, and know when to seek help from a medical professional.

When cells grow in an excessive or uncontrolled way, as cancer cells do, they form a lump or mass. Doctors call this lump a *tumor*. The most common sign of breast cancer is the presence of a lump in the breast, which the patient feels as being different from the rest of her breast.

If you ever feel anything in your breast that feels like your knuckle—round, discrete, and harder than normal—go to see your doctor right away. That's a bit of an exaggeration, because rarely is the lump as hard as a bony knuckle. But it is firmer than normal breast tissue.

It is very important to stress that sometimes the lump isn't so obvious, and there may simply be a vague area of firmness, rather than a discrete lump or mass. This is especially true of a specific type of breast cancer called *invasive lobular cancer*.

If the area in question in the breast feels different from the rest of the breast and the corresponding area in the other breast, go to see a doctor right away.

If a "different" feeling in your breast can be important, it stands to reason that every woman should become familiar with how her breasts feel at different times in her menstrual cycle. Any change from the norm should be a cause for concern and needs to be investigated.

Sometimes cancer may cause discomfort or even pain in the breast, and this may be the first sign that something is wrong. I am not talking about the pain or discomfort that many women experience just before menstruation. That is usually felt in both breasts in a symmetrical way,

Signs of Breast Cancer

- A lump or area of thickening

- An area of pain or tenderness

- An itchy rash on the nipple or areola

- Dimpling of the skin of the breast and/or nipple retraction

- A persistent discharge from one nipple, especially if it is bloodstained or colored

- Diffuse redness of the skin of the breast, especially if one breast feels heavier than the other

- The first sign of cancer in the breast may be due to a secondary cancer (metastasis) in the armpit or at a more distant site, such as bone or in the abdomen.

- Sometimes there may be no signs at all.

usually affects the upper-outer areas of both breasts, is most common a few days before the period, and generally disappears after the first day or two of starting menstrual flow.

What is much more sinister is pain or tenderness in one area of a breast that persists for several weeks. Postmenopausal women should not experience pain or tenderness in the breast unless they are taking hormone (estrogen) replacement therapy.

Other less common signs of cancer include a dimpling of the skin, retraction of the nipple, or the discharge of fluid from the nipple, especially if the fluid is bloodstained.

In some rare cases, the first sign of cancer may be the development of a red rash in the skin of the breast. This is sometimes associated with pain, tenderness, and diffuse thickening of the skin of the breast that takes on an orange-peel appearance with numerous little pits. This can look quite like inflammation due to an infection, so this kind of cancer is called *inflammatory breast cancer.*

In a small number of patients (no more than 5 percent of all patients with breast cancer), the first sign of breast cancer may actually be due to spread of the cancer from the breast to a distant site such as bone. This is a process called *metastases* and is less commonly the first sign of breast cancer than with diseases, such as lung cancer or cancer of the pancreas.

Bottom line: Pay attention to your body, and don't delay in seeing a physician if you feel something unusual in your breast.

CHAPTER 2

Staging and Biology
of Breast Cancer

*"Receiving a breast cancer diagnosis brought my life to an abrupt halt.
I experienced panic, anxiety, and contemplated certain death, since that is what
the word 'cancer' meant to me at the time."*
—*Terrece Crawford*

As a doctor who treats patients with breast cancer every day, I am constantly evaluating the important factors that determine the prognosis and treatment required to provide the very best chance of cure for each and every patient. No one can give you meaningful advice specific to your situation unless he or she knows all the details of your particular case.

It is very important for patients with breast cancer to recognize that, just as no two people are exactly the same, no two cancers are exactly the same. Please keep this in mind when friends and family give well-meaning advice: other people's stories and experiences may be completely irrelevant to your own situation.

When evaluating a patient with newly diagnosed breast cancer, we consider two important factors: the stage and the biology of the disease. Both of these have an important bearing on the ultimate prognosis for the patient and also on the treatment that we will recommend.

Staging is the process of understanding how much cancer is present and where it resides. There are several internationally recognized systems for staging breast cancer based on three elements:

- the **size** of the primary tumor in the breast;
- the presence or absence of cancer in the **lymph nodes** of the axilla; and
- the presence or absence of cancer in **distant sites,** such as liver, bone, lung, or brain. (We call spread to other organs **distant metastases.**)

Because the breast is a superficial organ (located near the surface of the body), a tumor in the breast is generally easy to feel. So, unlike cancer of the lung, pancreas, or prostate, where the tumor is buried deep in the body, most breast cancers can be diagnosed at an early stage.

What is the relevance of stage to prognosis and treatment?

These three elements are often combined in stage groupings, described below in a simplified fashion:

Stage 0: DCIS only, no invasive cancer. Almost always curable.

Stage I: Small tumor in breast only (less than two centimeters in diameter), no lymph node involvement. Typically treated with surgery and radiation. Some may have chemotherapy. High probability of cure.

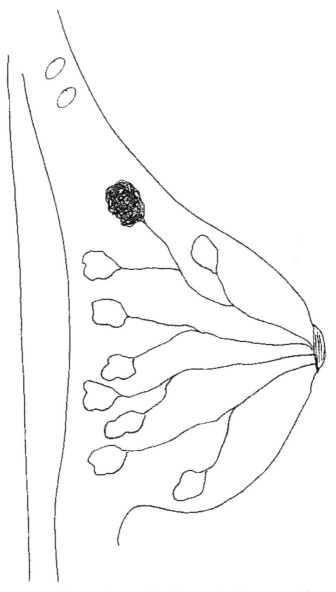

Stage I Breast Cancer. Small tumor in the breast with no spread to armpit (axillary) lymph nodes.

Stage II: Larger tumor in breast (two to five centimeters in diameter) and/or lymph node involvement. Typically treated with surgery and radiation. Most may have chemotherapy. Moderate probability of cure.

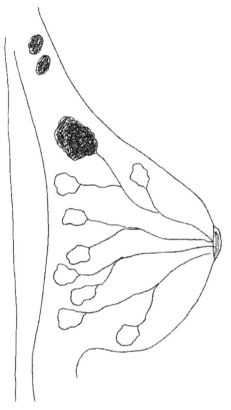

Stage II Breast Cancer. Larger tumor in the breast with disease spread to armpit (axillary) lymph nodes.

Stage III: Very large tumor in breast (greater than five centimeters in diameter) or extensive lymph-node involvement. Generally requires chemotherapy before surgery and will also require radiation. Some patients with Stage III disease may be cured, and with proper treatment, many Stage III patients can live for many years with an excellent quality of life.

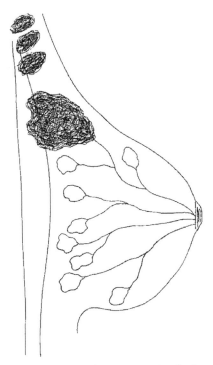

Stage III Breast Cancer. Very large tumor in the breast invading the muscle of the chest wall, extensive involvement of the lymph nodes.

Stage IV: Any size tumor in breast and lymph node with spread to distant organs. Complete cure is rarely a realistic goal in such patients. Patients are treated to extend their lives (often for years) and also to give the very best possible quality of life by relieving symptoms and preventing complications from the cancer.

Even in patients with widespread metastatic disease, there may be benefits to surgically removing the primary cancer by surgically removing all or part of the affected breast.

What is biologic typing of cancer?

Staging answers the question of *how much* cancer is present and exactly where the cancer is located. Biologic typing determines *what type* of cancer is present. Both stage and biology have an important influence on prognosis and treatment.

Over the past twenty years, we have learned a great deal about breast cancer biology and how it affects treatment choices. No two people are exactly alike, and the same is true of cancers. Some cancers are nastier than others. They are more aggressive, grow more quickly, spread to other tissues faster, and cause much more trouble for neighboring tissue and organs.

Important Biological Factors of Breast Cancer

Tumor grade

Estrogen and Progesterone receptor (ER/PR)

HER2neu

Ki67

Gene structure (onco*type* DX® and MammaPrint®)

Tumor Grade

Broadly speaking, tumor grade describes how the cancer *looks* under the microscope. It describes the general architecture of the cancer tissue and also the individual cells. Some cancers are rather bland looking, and others look mean and ugly.

The appearance of breast cancers is graded on a scale of one to three. Grade one indicates cancers that look something like normal breast tissue, while grade three are the mean-looking tumors. Knowing the grade of a specific breast cancer gives doctors an important clue to their future behavior. The higher the grade of the cancer, the more aggressive the tumor is likely to be and the poorer the prognosis is for the patient.

Estrogen and Progesterone Receptors (ER/PR)

Normal breast cells are sensitive to the effects of female sex hormones, particularly estrogen. Simply stated, estrogen makes breast cells grow. That is why young girls' breasts grow when they reach puberty and why most women experience some breast tenderness and discomfort just before their periods.

How is it that a hormone produced in the ovary can affect the cells in the breast? Well, in common with many other chemicals, the estrogen that a woman produces in her ovary is carried through the blood and ultimately comes into very close contact with the cells in the ducts of the breast (and many other tissues of the body).

All estrogen-sensitive cells contain an estrogen-binding protein. We call this protein Estrogen Binding Protein or Estrogen Receptor (often called ER for short). All normal breast cells contain this receptor. Estrogen binds to the cell through the estrogen receptor, and that is what stimulates the breast cell to divide.

Some breast cancer cells can also be shown to contain high levels of ER. And those breast cancer cells that contain ER are stimulated to grow by estrogen.

Like a key fitting into a lock, the binding of estrogen and the estrogen receptor is very specific, and when estrogen binds to the receptor, the cell is switched on and stimulated to grow.

Generally speaking, ER-positive breast cancers contain cells that more closely resemble normal breast cells. They are biologically less aggressive, meaning they grow more slowly and are less likely to spread early than ER-negative breast cancers.

It has been recognized for many years that ER-positive breast cancers carry a better prognosis than ER-negative breast cancers. When similar stage cancers are compared, patients with ER-positive cancers have almost 10 percent higher cure rates than patients with ER-negative disease.

Estrogen Receptor

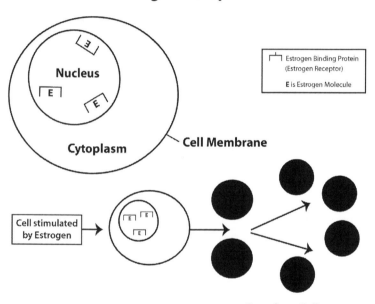

Daughter Cells

Another advantage of having an ER-positive breast cancer is that we have additional weapons to use to fight against this type of cancer, namely **hormone-blocking therapy**.

Progesterone binding protein (Progesterone Receptor or PR) is similar, but biologically and clinically less important than ER.

HER2neu

HER2neu is one of a family of four proteins called Epidermal Growth Factor Receptors present in some cancers. These proteins can influence tumor cell growth and spread (metastasis). Approximately 20 percent of breast cancers can be shown to contain the protein called HER2neu.

HER2neu was recognized about ten years ago to be a biologic factor of great importance in breast cancer. Finding HER2neu is kind of a bad news/good news discovery. The bad news is that HER2neu-positive breast cancers are faster growing and more likely to spread.

The good news is that there are several drugs available that specifically target the HER2neu protein and offer very effective treatment for patients with HER2neu-positive breast cancer. The first of these drugs to be approved was trastuzumab.

Trastuzumab is used very effectively to treat patients with advanced HER2neu-positive breast cancer. It also is used to prevent recurrence of the disease after breast cancer surgery (more about this adjuvant treatment in Chapter 7).

It is no exaggeration to say that the recognition of the HER2neu protein and the drugs used to attack it are among the biggest advances in breast cancer treatment in the last twenty years.

Ki67

Cancer grows through cell division. We now have the ability to accurately measure how active that cell division really is by measuring how many cells in cancer tissue are actively dividing. This is expressed as the Ki67 score: the higher the value of Ki67, the more actively the cells are dividing. Using Ki67 scoring, we can identify fast-growing cancers that often will require more aggressive treatment.

A high Ki67 score is seen most often in ER-negative cancers and indicates a rapidly growing cancer. These cancers require chemotherapy (as opposed to hormone treatment) but are more likely to be sensitive to drug treatment.

Breast Cancer Genomics

Each human cell contains genes—complex chemicals that allow the cell to produce an exact copy of itself, or in other words, to reproduce. Everyone has heard of DNA and RNA, the chemicals that form the basis of genetics.

Genetics is the study of how inherited traits are passed from one generation to the next through the genes, and how new traits appear by way of genetic mutations or changes. An increased risk of developing breast cancer may be inherited through an inherited mutation in the BRCA1 or BRCA2 gene, which we will discuss in detail later.

Breast cancer genomics is the study of the gene structure of breast cancer cells. Genomic tests identify specific genes present in the cancer cell and provide valuable information to help develop specific treatment plans for each patient.

There are now available relatively inexpensive genomic tests that your doctor can order to provide valuable information about your cancer. These tests can be performed on a simple biopsy specimen and are generally covered by medical insurance.

Based on genomic studies, we now recognize that breast cancer is not a single disease entity. Rather there is a spectrum of diseases, which require different treatment plans. Gene profiling has identified four major subtypes of breast cancer: Luminal A, Luminal B, Basal, and HER2 positive.

Genomic tests provide a level of accuracy and sophistication far beyond what was available even ten years ago. We can use this

How Genomic Studies Are Changing Breast Cancer Treatment

Prognosis: more accurate prediction of future course allows us to identify those patients who need (and those who do not need) drug treatment after surgery.

Molecular Subtype: more accurate characterization of the type of breast cancer, which affects prognosis and drug treatment.

Specific Cellular Targets for Treatment: established targets are estrogen receptor (endocrine therapy) and HER2neu (herceptin and related drugs).

Specific Gene Mutations: that may represent specific targets for new drugs in the future.

information to predict prognosis, whether a patient with early stage breast cancer is at low or high risk of future relapse. Based on this, we can better determine whether she needs drug (chemotherapy) treatment to improve her chance of cure.

We previously described the HER2neu gene and the specific drugs, like trastuzumab, which specifically targets it or the proteins derived from it. This has provided the basis for some of the most effective treatments for breast cancer over the past twenty years.

There is a great deal of research being done using genomic studies to identify additional gene mutations that may act to drive particular cancers. The identification of a specific gene in a cancer offers the opportunity to treat the cancer with a drug that specifically targets that gene. This offers the potential for more effective and less toxic treatment.

Breast cancer genomics already offer us the promise of more accurate diagnosis and more effective treatment. Molecular subtyping of breast cancer is a new technology, which has great potential, and these tests are likely to be used much more frequently in the future.

Clinical Significance of Tumor Biology

The biologic factors that we have just described provide doctors with useful information about how aggressive a particular tumor is likely to be. Your doctor will have a good idea of your *prognosis* (probability of a future good result, or the opposite) from this information.

Simply stated, a patient with a good prognosis tumor will need less aggressive medical treatment than a patient whose tumor has a less favorable prognostic profile.

For example, it is well established that ER-positive cancers generally have a better prognosis than ER-negative tumors. There are, however, approximately 30 percent of ER-positive cancers that represent a more aggressive form of the disease.

These are the 30 percent of ER patients who will suffer a relapse of their disease, despite being diagnosed at an early stage with relatively small tumors and negative lymph nodes. The challenge has always been to identify those ER-positive patients who are more likely to relapse and therefore need more aggressive treatment (generally chemotherapy).

It is important to emphasize that the biologic differences have little or no impact on the *local treatment* that is recommended. Put another way, the same principles of surgical and radiation treatment apply to all patients with early stage breast cancer.

The importance of biology is in identifying different prognosis (chance of cure) for different cancers and identifying the different *drug treatments* needed to prevent recurrence and achieve cure.

Combining Stage and Biology to Predict Outcome and Determine Treatment

All of the important factors discussed in this chapter are evaluated in every patient newly diagnosed with breast cancer to produce a clear picture of the patient's prognosis. It is the responsibility of the treating oncologist to incorporate all staging and biologic information into a coherent treatment plan that is highly individualized for each patient. See the accompanying table for all relevant factors.

Every patient with breast cancer should be fully informed regarding the stage and biology of her disease. All of this information should be known before any treatment is started.

There has been a paradigm shift in recent years in how we treat the breast cancer patient.

The old way of doing business, in which a general surgeon would immediately perform a mastectomy after a positive diagnosis and then refer the patient to a medical oncologist, is obsolete. All women with breast cancer deserve the benefit of the combined expertise of knowledgeable experts in all fields of cancer medicine—surgery, radiation, and medical oncology—*before* treatment is initiated so that they can fully benefit from all of the advances that have occurred in the past twenty years.

Today, the modern approach is to obtain all relevant information regarding the stage of the disease and biology (including genomics) before implementing a multidisciplinary treatment. Surgery is often not the first step in treatment.

Important Prognostic Factors in a Patient with Early Breast Cancer

	Favorable	Intermediate	Unfavorable
Tumor Factors			
STAGE			
Size of invasive tumor	0–1 cm	1–2 cm	>2 cm
Status of lymph nodes	negative	1–3 positive	>3 positive
BIOLOGY			
Grade	1	2	3
ER/PR	positive		negative
HER2neu	negative		positive
Ki67	Low	Intermediate	High
Molecular Subtype	Luminal A	Luminal B	Basal, HER2 positive
oncotype DX®	<18	19–30	>31
MammaPrint®	low risk		high risk
PATIENT FACTORS			
Age	>50	40–50	<40
Comorbidities	absent		present
Patient compliance	high		low

CHAPTER 3

Can Breast Cancer
Be Prevented?

"If I hadn't gone for the mammogram,
I would never have known there was a problem."
—Candace Fulsher

Some cancers have clear, well-defined causes. The best example is cigarette smoking and its relationship to lung cancer. But there are plenty of other cause/effect cancers, such as hepatitis C and liver cancer; asbestos exposure and mesothelioma; human papilloma virus and cancer of the cervix; radiation and some forms of leukemia; excessive ultraviolet radiation and skin cancer; and exposure to certain organic chemicals and bladder cancer.

When the cause of a cancer has been clearly identified by epidemiologic study (the study of large populations to identify the causes of disease), it is relatively easy in theory to prevent the cancer from occurring. Simply avoid exposure to the causative agent, and the disease is much less likely to occur.

Unfortunately, there is no single factor identified as *the* cause of breast cancer. It is certainly not like lung cancer, where avoiding tobacco has resulted in a major reduction in the incidence of the disease.

But there are some factors that do increase the risk for developing breast cancer (see page 44). If there is any single unifying concept that explains the development of breast cancer, it appears to be excessive stimulation of cells within the breast by the female sex hormone estrogen, whether produced naturally or given to women to treat or prevent symptoms or complications of menopause (such as hot flashes or thinning of the bones, known as *osteoporosis*). The other important factor that has been clearly established to increase breast cancer risk is a gene mutation known as BRCA.

Studies show that the majority of women who develop breast cancer do not have evidence of estrogen excess. So in these patients, we don't know why they develop breast cancer. Is their breast tissue simply more sensitive to estrogen stimulation, or is some other factor at work? We just don't know.

Since the medical community cannot identify a specific cause for breast cancer yet, we must instead focus on those things that we can control—early detection and prompt and appropriate treatment.

Primary Prevention

If you receive a flu shot, you likely won't come down with the flu. If you lower your blood pressure and cholesterol, you'll be much less likely to have a heart attack or stroke. These are methods of primary prevention. What follows are a few examples of primary prevention for breast cancer.

Prophylactic Mastectomy

The only completely effective primary prevention of breast cancer involves surgically removing both breasts (*prophylactic mastectomy*). A clearly radical approach, prophylactic removal of both breasts should only be considered if the lifetime risk of developing breast cancer is very high.

Medical Conditions Where Prophylactic Mastectomy Should Be Considered

- BRCA gene mutation (or other gene mutations which greatly increase breast cancer risk)

- Strong family history without gene mutation (e.g., multiple relatives with breast cancer in different generations, bilateral breast cancer, male breast cancer, breast cancer at very young age)

- Previous radiation treatment to chest in adolescence or young adult (usually for Hodgkin Disease)

- Previous breast biopsy showed high-risk changes

Numerous studies have shown that many woman will have an exaggerated idea of what their true risk is. I strongly recommend that before any woman takes the irreversible step of undergoing prophylactic bilateral mastectomy, she should consult a breast cancer specialist and a genetics counselor (where appropriate) so that she has a very clear idea of what her lifetime risk for developing breast cancer really is.

Every woman should also meet with a reconstructive (plastic) surgeon before mastectomy so that she understands exactly what her options are for breast reconstruction.

Prophylactic Oophorectomy

Surgical removal of the ovaries (the source of the majority of the body's estrogen) in premenopausal women significantly reduces the risk of developing breast cancer. Removing the ovaries, however, has serious effects on fertility and sexuality. Although the removal of the ovaries may be recommended as part of the treatment of breast cancer, it is only recommended to prevent breast cancer in women with a very high risk for developing breast cancer, such as women with a BRCA gene mutation.

Reduce Estrogen

It is clear that estrogen stimulates the growth of normal breast cells, and we know that whenever cells are stimulated to grow, there is a potential for serious damage to occur in the DNA content of the cell. Repeated DNA damage over a prolonged period of time eventually may lead to the development of cancer.

Risk Factors for Developing Breast Cancer

- Gene mutations (BRCA and others)
- Family history of breast or ovarian cancer
- Previous history of breast cancer
- Reproductive factors: early onset of periods, late menopause, no full-term pregnancies
- History of estrogen therapy
- History of radiation to neck or chest as child or young adult (e.g., for Hodgkin Disease)
- Lifestyle factors
- Fibrocystic disease of the breast with abnormal cells present (doctors refer to this as Atypical Ductal Hyperplasia or ADH)
- Lobular Carcinoma in Situ (LCIS)

We have known for many years that women treated after menopause with a combination of estrogen and progesterone have an increased risk of developing breast cancer. A major study completed in 2002, the Women's Health Initiative, confirmed this increased risk, and the International Agency for Research on Cancer now classifies this combination of estrogen and progesterone as a human carcinogen (a cancer-causing agent).

Many of the reproductive, lifestyle, and dietary factors known to increase breast cancer risk also have the effect of increasing estrogen stimulation of breast cells (see table).

Lifestyle Factors That Contribute to Breast Cancer: Obesity, Exercise, and Diet

Studies have shown that obesity and lack of physical activity increase the risk for developing breast cancer. Research has also shown that obesity has an important effect on the *prognosis* of women who have been diagnosed with breast cancer. In other words, obese women with breast cancer are more likely to die of their disease than non-obese women.

Before the link between breast cancer and obesity was studied, doctors used to think that obese women were more apt to develop advanced-stage disease due to difficulties in detecting the breast cancer. However, thanks to clinical studies on the topics of obesity and breast cancer, several other reasons have recently been suggested for the poorer prognosis in obese women.

First, overweight women are more likely to be diagnosed with triple-negative breast cancer, which has more limited treatment options (we will discuss triple-negative breast cancer in Chapter 14).

Second, it is known that Aromatase Inhibitors, an important class of drugs that reduce estrogen levels, are less effective in treating breast cancer in obese patients. Obese women have lower levels of a protein called Sex Hormone Binding Globulan (SHBG), so their blood levels of free (active) estrogen are higher than women who are not obese.

Studies show that both a low calorie diet and moderate to vigorous exercise will lower estrogen levels. But it is not necessary for women to exercise at an intense level to protect themselves from breast cancer. Regular moderate exercise not only reduces breast cancer risk, but also reduces the risk of cancer recurrence following treatment.

A recent Italian study of five thousand women (twenty-five hundred patients with breast cancer and the same number of control subjects) published in the *Journal of the National Cancer Institute* estimated that about one-third of breast cancer cases can be attributed to nutrition and physical exercise. A diet rich in vegetables and fruits is associated with a reduced breast cancer risk, while a diet high in animal fat (particularly dairy products) is associated with higher risk.

It should be noted, though, that studies of extremely low-fat diets have produced disappointing results, in that they have so far failed to reduce breast cancer incidence.

Alcohol

It has been clearly established that regular alcohol consumption increases the risk of developing breast cancer, with **a direct relationship between the amount of alcohol consumed on a regular basis and the level of increased risk.** Several studies have shown that alcohol administration increases blood estrogen levels.

Recently, the Million Women Study in the United Kingdom reported that even one alcoholic drink per day increases a woman's cancer risk. The authors of this study estimate that as many as 11 percent of breast cancers may be directly due to alcohol. They concluded that, as far as breast cancer is concerned, "There is no level of alcohol consumption that can be considered safe."

Smoking

Although breast cancer is not usually thought of as one of the cancers closely associated with cigarette smoking, there is some evidence to support an association between the two.

A recent report from the University of Pittsburgh followed thirteen thousand patients in the NSABP Breast Cancer Prevention Trial. Study results showed a much higher risk of invasive breast cancer in smokers than in nonsmokers. Women who smoked for more than thirty-five years had a 60 percent higher risk of breast cancer than women who never smoked. Women who smoked for less than fifteen years had no increased risk of breast cancer.

Measures to Reduce Breast Cancer Risk

There are simple lifestyle changes that any woman can make that also will help reduce her risk of developing breast cancer:

- Eat a diet low in animal fat.
- Get regular physical exercise.
- Keep your weight down.
- Drink very little alcohol, if at all.
- Avoid cigarettes completely.
- Get adequate amounts of vitamin D and calcium, which may also help reduce breast cancer risk.

Another study (from Yale University) of 796 women with early-stage breast cancer who smoked showed that the risk of developing a second cancer of the breast was greater in smokers when compared to nonsmokers (25 percent compared with 19 percent).

All of these studies suggest that women who adopt healthy lifestyles will significantly reduce their risk for developing breast cancer. Additionally, making healthy choices will benefit women who have already been diagnosed and treated for breast cancer.

Drug Treatment with Selective Estrogen Receptor Modulators

Just as treatment with estrogen increases the risk for developing breast cancer, treatment that reduces the effect of estrogen also **reduces the risk** of developing breast cancer. Many of the estrogen-reducing treatments for breast cancer also are effective when used to reduce the risk of developing the disease and can therefore be used to prevent breast cancer.

There are now prescription drugs available that reduce the stimulatory effect of estrogen on the breast. Known as SERMS (Selective Estrogen Receptor Modulators), these drugs include tamoxifen and raloxifene.

Tamoxifen has been used effectively and safely for approximately forty years to treat women with breast cancer. Tamoxifen is also helpful in reducing the risk of a second cancer from developing in the opposite (unaffected) breast. Studies have shown that women at high risk of developing breast cancer who took tamoxifen for five years reduced their risk of developing cancer by approximately 40 percent. It is important to note that the reduced risk for developing breast cancer continued even after the drug was stopped.

Although tamoxifen is an estrogen-blocking drug as far as the breast is concerned, it has estrogen-like activity on other tissues, including the uterus. As a result, prolonged use of tamoxifen slightly increases the risk for developing cancer of the lining of the uterus (endometrial cancer).

As with any drug, it is important to put the risk of serious side effects of tamoxifen into perspective. In the NSABP P-1 study, which demonstrated a positive reduction in breast cancer incidence due to tamoxifen, women were approximately twice as likely to develop uterine (endometrial) cancer as those who received an inactive placebo (the control group). Most of these uterine cancers are cured by hysterectomy (surgical removal of the uterus).

Raloxifene

Raloxifene is another SERM used primarily to treat and prevent osteoporosis. In a head-to-head comparison with tamoxifen, raloxifene was slightly less effective in preventing breast cancer (23 percent vs 38 percent). But raloxifene was associated with fewer severe side effects, such as blood clots and uterine cancer, when compared with tamoxifen.

It should be noted that SERMS are effective at preventing ER-positive breast cancer but do not appear to reduce the risk of ER-negative breast cancer.

Having said this, both tamoxifen and raloxifene are approved by the FDA for the primary prevention of breast cancer in high-risk women. Many women are reluctant to take these drugs because of concerns about side effects. But in many cases, the risk of serious side effects is far outweighed by the benefits in terms of reduction in cancer incidence.

If you have one or more of the risk factors listed on page 44, you should discuss with your doctor whether you may be a candidate for an estrogen blocking or lowering drug.

Secondary Prevention: Early Diagnosis

It is no exaggeration to say that every woman should consider herself at risk for developing breast cancer. That's why secondary prevention through early diagnosis and tertiary prevention through prompt and appropriate treatment are so important.

Secondary prevention refers to improving the chances of complete cure of breast cancer through diagnosis of the disease at the earliest possible moment, and the earliest possible stage.

This is a very realistic goal for two reasons. First, unlike many cancers, such as those of the lung, pancreas, stomach and ovary, cancer of the breast occurs in an organ that is very close to the surface of the body. Cancerous tumors that develop in organs deep within the body can grow to a relatively large size and spread to many distant areas of the body before they produce any symptoms to make the patient aware that anything is wrong.

In contrast, breast cancer usually forms a lump in the breast that can be felt by the patient and the doctor. So diagnosis can be made relatively early in the course of the disease. Additionally, we can now identify cancers when they are still very tiny, long before they can be felt through the use of screening mammography.

Screening Mammograms Save Lives

There are two rules that every woman should heed: Once a woman reaches forty years of age, she should have a screening mammogram every year. And if she suspects that something is wrong with one or both of her breasts, she shouldn't delay. She should go to a doctor who specializes in breast diseases.

It is critically important to diagnose breast cancer at the very earliest possible moment, preferably long before it has become large enough to produce a lump or any other sign in the breast. That's what screening mammograms are all about.

A mammogram is an X-ray picture of the breast. It is now well recognized that many women may have breast cancer visible on their mammograms years before they have any signs of breast cancer or any palpable lump. It can appear as a tiny mass, an area of distortion of the usual pattern of normal breast tissue, or as a cluster of tiny calcium deposits.

There are two basic types of mammograms: a *screening* mammogram and a *diagnostic* mammogram.

A diagnostic mammogram is an X-ray study of a particular area of the breast and is ordered if a woman feels a lump or has some other symptom that draws attention to an area of the breast. A diagnostic mammogram may also be ordered if a screening mammogram has shown an abnormality.

We will discuss diagnostic mammograms in further detail in the next chapter when we discuss tools for diagnosing breast cancer.

Screening Mammograms

Screening for any particular disease means looking at large numbers of people who feel 100 percent fine to identify those people who have the very earliest stage of that disease at a time when it is still completely curable. Examples of screening include getting a PAP smear to diagnose early cancer of the cervix or having your blood pressure or cholesterol checked.

The goal is to screen the entire female population who are at risk for developing breast cancer, and the best way to do that is through annual screening mammograms.

Although there is some debate over whether women should have their first screening mammogram beginning at age forty, and whether screening mammograms should be every year or every two years, everyone agrees that certainly after age fifty every woman should have regular mammograms **no matter how her breasts feel.**

The screening mammogram involves taking two complete X-ray images of each breast: an up-and-down view (known as CC, cranio-caudad, or head to tail) and a side-to-side view (known as MLO, or medio-lateral oblique). Doctors are looking for any area of the breast that looks different from the way it appeared on a previous mammogram or that looks different from the corresponding area in the opposite breast. The radiologist reading the film looks for areas of increased density, asymmetry, or clustered microcalcifications. If such an area is seen on a screening mammogram, then the next step is usually to order a diagnostic mammogram.

Mammograms can show a cancer in the breast long before anything abnormal can be felt. Most breast cancers can't be felt until they are about one centimeter (approximately half an inch) in diameter. But a screening mammogram can allow diagnosis of a cancer when it is only a few millimeters in size.

Numerous studies have clearly demonstrated that women who have regular screening mammograms have their cancers diagnosed at an earlier stage (with a smaller tumor in the breast and less chance of axillary nodes involved) and, as a result, have a lower death rate from breast cancer.

The Debate about Mammograms

Despite these facts, there is still a continued debate among medical doctors about the value of regular screening mammograms in women who feel nothing wrong with their breasts.

Critics of the practice are correct when they say that having a normal mammogram doesn't guarantee that a woman can't or won't develop breast cancer in the future. And it is also true that mammograms tend to identify the slower-growing and less aggressive types of breast cancer, while some of the more aggressive breast cancers may not be seen on a routine mammogram, especially in younger women.

There is also a risk of false positive results—mammogram results that raise the possibility of cancer, cause major anxiety for the patient, and possibly lead to an unnecessary biopsy when, in fact, no cancer is present.

Another argument is that regular screening mammograms may lead to an overdiagnosis of breast cancer by identifying more women with preinvasive cancer changes in the breast (the DCIS described earlier). Critics of screening mammograms argue that many of these cases of DCIS would never have become invasive cancer.

Another concern regarding mammograms is that, since they are X-ray studies and result in radiation exposure, they could increase the risk for developing cancer. This is more of a theoretical than practical concern because the number of breast cancers *caused* by mammograms is estimated to be tiny. It is estimated that approximately sixty women develop breast cancer attributable to mammograms every year in the United States, compared to the thousands of lives saved every year by screening mammograms.

In my opinion, the arguments against mammographic screening are hard to support for the following reasons:

- The overwhelming majority of scientific studies show that women who have regular mammographic screenings for breast cancer are diagnosed at an earlier stage. As a result, the death rate from breast cancer is lowered by approximately 25 percent.
- A patient with a tiny screen-detected cancer is much more likely to be successfully treated and cured when compared with a woman with a large palpable lump. Not only is she more likely to be cured, but the treatment needed to achieve that cure is likely to be much easier and more tolerable.

For all of these reasons, most authorities, including the American Cancer Society (ACS) and the National Cancer Institute (NCI), recommend regular screening mammograms in healthy women.

Should you start routine mammogram screenings at forty or fifty?

Overall, there is no doubt that women age fifty and older should have regular mammographic screenings. There is, however, considerable debate whether women between forty and fifty should have annual screenings for the following reasons:

- Those who argue against screening this age group point out that the risk for breast cancer in women aged forty to fifty is relatively small, so the probability of a positive mammogram is relatively small.
- Although less women will develop breast cancer between the ages of forty and forty-nine, the risk is not negligible. One in sixty-nine develop breast cancer during the ten years between ages forty and fifty, compared to one in forty-two women aged fifty to sixty, and one in twenty-nine women aged sixty to seventy.
- Another argument states that mammograms are less sensitive in younger women who are still menstruating regularly. Normal breast

tissue appears denser on the mammogram film, and may obscure an early cancer.

- While this is true, a mammogram is still a very useful screening test. The strongest argument in favor of screening younger women is the fact, established by large clinical studies, that there is a 15 percent reduction in the breast cancer death rate in women aged forty to fifty who have regular screening mammograms when compared with an unscreened population.
- Another argument against mammograms in women aged forty to fifty relates to the risk of unnecessary biopsies because of a false positive mammogram. It is estimated that approximately 30 percent will have a false positive mammogram during ages forty to fifty, and that 7 percent to 8 percent will have a breast biopsy. But know that breast biopsies can be accomplished by a very simple nonsurgical technique (described in more detail in the next chapter).

I have personally treated hundreds of younger women with breast cancer, many whose diagnoses were made by screening mammograms long before they would have been able to feel a breast lump. In forty years of medical practice, I've never heard a woman complain after being told that her breast biopsy was negative and that she didn't have cancer. Each reaction was always one of relief.

As a physician specializing in breast cancer, it is my opinion that every woman aged forty and older should have an annual screening mammogram because the benefits far outweigh the risks.

Every day, I see about a dozen women with breast cancer. Some of them are diagnosed through screening mammograms. But in far too many cases, the patient isn't diagnosed until she feels a lump. And sometimes it is a big lump. When I ask the patient, "Before this year, when was your last screening mammogram?" she will sometimes get a sheepish look and say something like, "Oh, five or six years ago."

This is not good. Not only are the cancers smaller when detected by screening mammograms, but they are much less likely to have spread beyond the breast. The cure rate for screen-detected cancers is much higher, and the treatment needed to achieve that cure is often much simpler.

Limitations of Mammograms

There are two important warnings associated with the screening mammogram. First, if you develop a lump in your breast after having a normal mammogram, you cannot assume that the lump is benign. You have to take it seriously. A negative mammogram three months ago does not mean that you can't have breast cancer. You must understand that, for every diagnostic test, there is a threshold of sensitivity below which the test will not identify an abnormality. The following analogy may be helpful to understanding the limitations of mammography:

Imagine you're sitting in a football stadium with one hundred thousand other people. You're looking for your friends, but you have no idea where they are sitting. How successful are you going to be in finding them? That's what a screening mammogram is intended to do—to find a tiny collection of cancer cells in a body that contains billions and billions of cells.

So the fact that a negative mammogram is not a 100 percent guarantee that you don't have an early breast cancer is just a limitation of the test itself.

Other limitations of mammograms include the following statements:

- Mammograms are less likely to show a tumor in very young women, or women who have been taking postmenopausal estrogen replacement, because the breast tissue appears denser on the X-ray film.
- Mammograms are also less sensitive with smaller tumors and the specific type of cancer called invasive lobular cancer.

The second warning is this: if you have a screening mammogram and don't hear from your doctor, **DO NOT ASSUME THAT EVERYTHING IS FINE.**

Doctors who read mammogram films can make mistakes. They can interpret the film incorrectly, and they can make the wrong recommendations based on their reading of the film. A mammogram is just a picture, and it is only as good as the guy who reads and interprets it.

Why Communication Is Critical

There are other, more subtle ways that screening mammograms can be rendered ineffective. Here's one example:

I recently saw a patient named Linda (not her real name), age fifty-three, who was newly diagnosed with breast cancer. Two-and-a-half years before I first saw her, she had a screening mammogram. At that time, she felt no lump in her breast, and the screening mammogram was interpreted as showing a mass that was thought to be of low probability for cancer. Based on that reading, the radiologist recommended a follow-up mammogram in six months.

This was the correct recommendation for Linda because the index of suspicion (meaning the probability that the abnormality was cancer) was so low that a repeat study in six months was appropriate.

Linda, like most people, was busy with other things in her life. Later on she told me, "I didn't go back in six months. The doctor had told me that it was probably a cyst, and I had a cyst on my ovary once. I knew that a cyst was no big deal."

Except it wasn't a cyst—it was cancer. I'm not critical of the doctor who read the film in 2007 and recommended a six-month follow up. And certainly Linda should have had the six-month follow up study that was recommended and should not have waited two years to have another screening mammogram.

I wondered if her actions would have been different if she'd been told this: "What we saw could be cancer. It's a low risk that it is cancer. If we judged it to be a high risk, we would recommend a biopsy immediately. But there is still a slight risk that it could be cancer. Please come back in six months, and we'll take another film. If it is only a cyst, it will either go away or won't change significantly. If we see any significant change in the repeat mammogram in six months, we'll arrange a biopsy at that time."

"If I had been told that," Linda told me, "then there is no way I would have put off the repeat study in six months."

Hindsight is twenty-twenty, but if the recommendation had been **communicated more effectively**, the patient would have paid more attention to it, and maybe the delay in diagnosis could have been avoided.

Because it is not just about reading the film correctly and making the correct recommendation. It is also about effectively communicating the results of the test and the recommendations that are derived from the test. Good doctors know how to communicate with people on a level they can understand.

(Update on Linda: Despite that long delay, Linda's cancer was not biologically aggressive, and did not significantly progress during that time. So when she became my patient, the cancer was still at a relatively early stage, and her prognosis for total cure remains very good.)

Here is another patient's story, but with a much less favorable outcome. A woman went for a screening mammogram that showed a highly suspicious nodule. The radiologist read the film correctly and recommended an immediate biopsy. The written report, with the recommendation for immediate biopsy, was sent to the patient's family doctor, where the report was promptly filed in the patient's chart. **None of the medical or nursing staff saw the report.**

The radiologist *assumed* that the family doctor was following the recommendation and was arranging a biopsy. And the patient *assumed* that the mammogram was fine because no one contacted her about it. No news is good news, right?

When she felt a lump in her breast six months later, she didn't worry because she knew that she had a negative mammogram six months earlier. Six months after that, the aggressive tumor in her breast had broken through the skin of the breast and had spread to her liver. And two years after that, she died.

In both of these stories, the doctors did nothing wrong. They read the mammograms correctly, and they made the correct recommendations. But in each case, there was a breakdown in communication.

There are lessons to be learned from these patient stories:

- It is not enough to have a screening mammogram each year.
- You need to know the result of your mammogram, and you have to follow the doctor's recommendations.
- Don't assume that no news is good news.
- Don't assume that a recent negative mammogram is any indication of current risk of cancer if you develop a breast lump shortly after the mammogram.
- When in doubt, check it out!

The Final Word about Screening Mammograms

I don't want to conclude this chapter on a negative note. Screening mammograms represent one of the major advances in breast cancer care of the last thirty years, and many thousands of women owe their lives to the simple fact that they went for a mammogram when they felt 100 percent fine.

DCIS is now diagnosed in approximately fifty thousand women every year in the United States, and this is largely because of screening mammograms.

We treat DCIS to prevent the future development of invasive breast cancer. When treated appropriately, almost all women with DCIS can be absolutely confident of complete cure.

Tertiary Prevention: Getting the Best Possible Treatment

Tertiary prevention is all about improving the chances of conquering breast cancer by making sure that patients diagnosed with breast cancer get the very best treatment available. And that process must begin with a good relationship between the doctor and the patient. The doctor must be committed to fully explaining the patient's condition and treatment options, to helping her navigate the health care system, and to helping her ultimately make the best treatment choices.

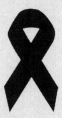

Screening Mammograms Detect Early Cancers

IN APRIL 2011, AT AGE FORTY-ONE, CANDACE FULSHER had her first screening mammogram. She had just lost her daughter in May 2010 to a lifelong battle with cancer and admits that she had put off taking care of herself to care for others.

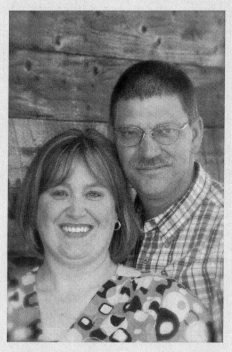

"If I had waited until I was fifty, like many doctors suggest, my cancer would likely have become invasive and much worse."
—Candace Fulsher, with her husband Mark

While her breasts felt fine, the mammogram showed a nodule (mass) in her left breast and tiny areas of calcification in both breasts.

Because of these findings on the mammogram, Candace had biopsies of both breasts. The biopsy of the right breast showed fibrocystic changes—a totally benign, noncancerous condition. But the biopsy of the left breast showed a tiny area of preinvasive cancer, DCIS (Ductal Carcinoma in Situ). The area was less than one inch in diameter.

"If I hadn't gone for a screening mammogram, I would never have known there was a problem," Candace says. "And if I had waited until I was fifty, like many doctors suggest, my cancer would likely have become invasive and much worse."

Following surgical removal of the area, Candace was treated with radiation to the left breast. She is taking tamoxifen to prevent any further development of DCIS or invasive cancer. When seen in November 2012, Candace was in excellent health with only mild discomfort in the left breast. She's committed to having annual screening mammograms.

Doctor's Comments

Candace's experience is very typical. Secondary prevention (early diagnosis) of breast cancer, often years before it ever becomes invasive, is now possible and is the direct result of screening mammography.

Approximately fifty thousand women are now diagnosed with DCIS every year. Treatment is relatively simple and very effective in preventing future development of invasive cancer.

CHAPTER 4

Tools for Diagnosing Breast Cancer

"I couldn't imagine why these doctors thought they were simple calcium deposits, given my extensive family history with cancer."
—*Deliz Santiago*

In the last chapter we discussed the importance of screening mammograms in women who don't suspect or feel anything wrong in their breasts. We're going to switch gears now and talk about what you should do if you *do* feel something abnormal in your breast.

Please see your doctor right away if you develop any of the danger signs listed in the table, *Signs of Breast Cancer,* on page 25. It is important to emphasize that cancer sometimes produces changes in the breast that are quite subtle, so if you have *any suspicion at all* that something's not right with your breast, don't ignore the problem. See your doctor.

I want to emphasize one other point, which is very important for younger women. Most women experience some discomfort in their breasts in the week or so before their period is due. The breasts of women who are still menstruating regularly are constantly changing because of the hormonal stimulation that occurs with their monthly cycle, **but if a lump persists through one or two menstrual cycles at most, it has to be considered as a possible cancer.**

In the same way, the breasts of women who are beyond menopause are no longer undergoing monthly changes due to hormonal stimulation. So if a postmenopausal woman develops a lump, chances are much higher that it is not fibrocystic disease, and that it could be cancerous. A postmenopausal woman with a significant breast lump needs to have it checked out by an experienced doctor without delay.

Examination is not enough.

Before discussing the various diagnostic tests that are available to investigate a breast lump, I have to make a very important point that relates to the limitations of the doctor's examination.

If you ever feel a lump in one breast and visit your doctor, do not be satisfied if your doctor examines your breasts and tells you that based on his or her examination, you don't have cancer and the lump you feel is due to fibrocystic disease.

It is a medical fact that **no doctor can tell with absolute certainty from physical examination alone that any lump is cancer or not.** He may become angry with you for questioning his clinical judgment. He may tell you that based on his years of clinical experience he *knows* it is not cancer. But the medical fact remains: no doctor can tell a benign lump from a malignant lump from his or her clinical examination alone. The doctor may have some basis for thinking that a lump is more likely to be noncancerous, but that's not 100 percent certain. Doctors may insist with great confidence that you don't have cancer based simply on their examination for several reasons:

First, fibrocystic disease is much more common than breast cancer in younger women. The average family doctor or gynecologist will see many more women with benign (noncancerous) breast lumps than women with breast cancer.

Second, medical students are taught early in their careers that the signs of cancer in the breast include skin dimpling, nipple retraction, skin nodules, and so on. These are the signs of *advanced* breast cancer. So in the woman who simply has a lump, the doctor who is not a specialist in breast diseases is more likely to think, "OK, I don't see any skin dimpling, nipple retraction, or skin nodules, so it must not be cancer."

But in patients with *early* breast cancer, the only sign that there is a problem is the presence of a lump. A single lump or mass that is freely mobile in the breast with no change in the skin certainly could be cancer. It could also be a benign (noncancerous) tumor, or it could be fibrocystic change. No doctor can tell with absolute certainty from feeling alone. And when there is a possibility of cancer, you want to know with absolute certainty.

If a doctor's examination is of limited value in diagnosing a breast lump, what diagnostic tools are available?

Diagnostic Mammograms

In contrast to a screening mammogram that looks at the entire breast, a diagnostic mammogram is an examination that focuses on a specific area in one breast or the other and is often done with magnification of the particular area of interest.

Your doctor may recommend a diagnostic mammogram either because the screening mammogram has shown a possible abnormality in a particular area, or you have some complaint—either a lump or pain and tenderness that has drawn attention to that area.

But be forewarned: A mammogram is NOT the final answer as to whether a lump in the breast is cancer. A mammogram is used to diagnose the cancer that you can't feel. It is not the first or most important test your doctor should order if you have a lump in the breast. This is a common error, and it is one that too many doctors still make.

A benign cyst and a malignant tumor can look very similar on a mammogram. You cannot tell them apart with a high degree of probability. So if your doctor says, "Good news, the mammogram showed that lump we feel is just a cyst," the doctor is flat-out WRONG. And you could be in real trouble.

I have personally reviewed the medical records of dozens of women in whom the diagnosis of breast cancer was needlessly delayed, often for many months and sometimes for years. Why? Because their doctors reassured them that the lumps they felt were not cancer, either based on their clinical examination, or because they didn't show up on the mammogram.

False Negative Mammograms

One of the most common mistakes that doctors make when investigating a woman who complains of a lump in her breast is to assume that if the mammogram shows no abnormality, then there is no cancer present. This is a major error.

We have known since the 1980s that a mammogram may fail to show an abnormality in some women who have a breast cancer that they and their doctors can feel as a palpable lump. There is, in medical terms, a definite *false negative rate* for mammograms in women with palpable breast cancer. This is particularly true in younger women (under the age of fifty), in women with smaller tumors, in women with lobular cancer of the breast, and in women whose breast tissue is denser than normal (due to younger age or estrogen-replacement therapy).

If you ask most doctors what the false negative rate is for mammograms in women with a palpable cancer, they will most likely tell you approximately 10 percent. In fact, in some studies reported in the 1980s, the false negative rate was 30 percent to 48 percent. Now, with modern digital mammograms, the false negative rate is probably much lower, **but it is still not zero.** So if you feel a lump, you cannot rely on a negative mammogram to exclude cancer.

So you may ask, "Why do a mammogram at all?" Well, we really order the mammogram to be sure the rest of the breast tissue is healthy and doesn't contain an impalpable cancer. It's important to remember that:

- you cannot rely on a negative mammogram to exclude cancer if you have a palpable mass;
- you cannot distinguish between a benign and malignant tumor from the appearance on a mammogram;
- if you have a palpable lump in your breast, you need an ultrasound examination of the area.

Ultrasound

Unlike the mammogram that looks at the entire breast, an ultrasound examination is focused on the problem area—in other words, on the lump itself. In an ultrasound exam, the technician or doctor bounces sound waves off that area in the breast, and the pattern of the ultrasound image helps suggest the correct diagnosis.

An ultrasound is the best way to distinguish between a *solid* mass (which means a tumor, either cancerous or benign) and a fluid-filled structure, called a *cyst*, which is much less likely to be cancerous. An ultrasound may provide one of three results:

- An ultrasound may tell your doctor that the lump is filled with fluid (in other words, that it is a cyst). There are basically two ways the cyst can appear on the ultrasound. If it is a *simple cyst*, with a thin wall, excellent transmission of the sound wave, and no internal echoes, then the risk of cancer is very low—no biopsy is needed. Your doctor may want to take the fluid out with a needle if it is causing you discomfort, but that's not a biopsy.
- The other possibility is that the ultrasound will show a *complex cyst*, meaning there is fluid visible, but there are some internal echoes. And the wall of the cyst is thicker with some irregularity to it. With a complex cyst, there is some risk of cancer, and a biopsy is recommended.
- The ultrasound may tell your doctor if the lump is *solid*, with no fluid in it. That's when the risk of cancer is high enough that an immediate biopsy is necessary.

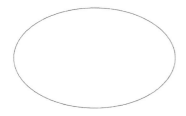

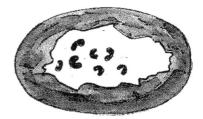

Simple cyst   *Complex cyst*

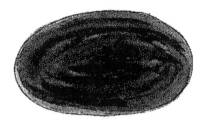

Solid tumor
Ultrasounds can distinguish between a simple cyst, a complex cyst, and a solid tumor.

Whenever the ultrasound examination shows a solid area or complex cyst, a *biopsy* is needed.

Biopsy

If you have a lump in your breast, the only way to make a definite diagnosis of cancer is by taking a tissue sample, or a biopsy.

In a biopsy, an actual sample of the breast tissue from the area in question is examined under a microscope. A biopsy is the only way to prove with almost 100 percent certainty* whether a lump, or other abnormality in the breast, is cancerous. In addition to establishing a cancer diagnosis, all of the important biological factors like grade, ER, HER2, and genomic studies that we discussed in Chapter 2 can also be determined from a core needle biopsy or limited surgical biopsy.

*On rare occasions, there may be doubts whether the breast tissue obtained at biopsy demonstrates cancer or not. This is a very uncommon occurrence, and any patient in this category will certainly be seeing a breast cancer specialist.

Is there any other way to make a diagnosis of cancer other than taking a biopsy? NO. If you have a lump in your breast and there is any serious possibility that this is cancer, you MUST have a biopsy.

Diagnostic Evaluation of Palpable Breast Mass

Physical Exam Confirms Mass

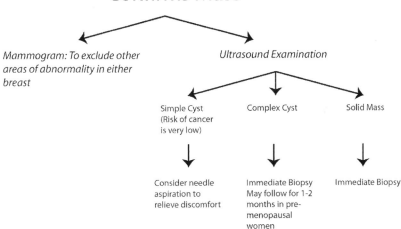

A woman beyond menopause who develops a firm, non-tender lump (an area that feels different from the rest of her breast) should consider the lump cancerous until proven otherwise. The patient MUST have a biopsy, without delay.

For a woman who is still having regular periods and feels something abnormal in one of her breasts, it is not unreasonable for her doctor to recommend that she wait for one or, at most, two menstrual cycles to see if the area in question disappears. In premenopausal woman, there is a higher probability that any palpable abnormality is due to fibrocystic change because of an hormonal effect on the breast.

However, in a premenopausal woman, if an ultrasound has shown the mass or lump to be solid (not cystic), then waiting to see if the mass disappears is NOT justified and immediate biopsy is needed, just as it is in a postmenopausal woman.

Sometimes a patient will tell a doctor that she doesn't want a biopsy because surgery will leave a big scar on her breast. This is not true. There are several ways to take a tissue sample without major surgery. The two most often used are **core needle biopsy** and **limited surgical excision.** Both are outpatient procedures that require local anesthesia only and will leave a minimal scar. More importantly, not only will each confirm the presence of cancer, but each will also provide additional information that allows your team of doctors to develop a complete treatment plan.

Magnetic Resonance Imaging (MRI)

MRI is a newer method of obtaining an image of the breast that uses a different technology from the X-ray. Although an MRI is more sensitive than the mammogram in detecting breast cancer, it is not yet so reliable that a biopsy can be avoided in patients with a mass that is suspicious for cancer.

One of the issues with MRI is that it may be too sensitive, meaning that minor abnormalities of no clinical significance may be frequently seen. The risk is that such false positive studies could lead to many unnecessary biopsies.

The major use of breast MRI is in evaluating the extent of disease in the breast when cancer has been diagnosed. It is possible that MRI may eventually have a role in the screening of women who are at particularly high risk for developing breast cancer (the patient with a BRCA mutation, for example), or in patients where mammography is of limited value (for example, patients with breast implants). At the moment, the precise role of breast MRI in screening the general population has not yet been defined.

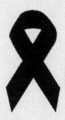

Every Lump Requires a Proper Diagnostic Evaluation

IN SEPTEMBER 2008, DELIZ SANTIAGO, age fifty-four, felt a lump in her left breast. Deliz works as a nurse in Joliet, Illinois, so she knew enough not to ignore it. She consulted her family doctor, who ordered a mammogram. The doctor told her that the mammogram showed "only calcification" and that no further action was needed.

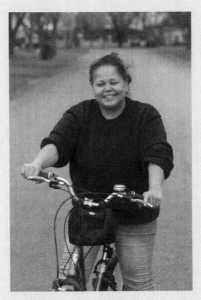

"Don't believe everything you hear. Get more opinions and seek the answers."
—Deliz Santiago

But Deliz has a significant family history of cancer. Her mother, her mother's sister (her maternal aunt), and her first cousin had all been diagnosed in the past with breast cancer.

"I couldn't imagine why these doctors thought these were simple calcium deposits, given my extensive family history," Deliz says.

Over the next few months, the lump continued to grow. She was concerned enough to speak to the doctor who works with her. He advised her to have further tests, and in February 2009, she had an ultrasound that revealed a solid mass. A biopsy confirmed that Deliz had invasive ER/PR-positive ductal carcinoma.

When Deliz then became my patient, the cancer in her left breast had grown to about six centimeters in diameter and had spread to her armpit lymph nodes.

Deliz received four cycles of chemotherapy with almost complete disappearance of the mass. Deliz then had a lumpectomy to remove the cancerous tumor in the breast and the affected lymph nodes. Following surgery, she received radiation therapy. When I last saw Deliz in June 2013, she remained cancer free. She is currently receiving five years of hormone (Aromatase Inhibitor) therapy.

"Women need to take charge of their health care and ask questions," Deliz cautions. "Don't believe everything you hear. Get more opinions and seek the answers."

Doctor's Comments

A mammogram is not the appropriate first diagnostic test for a woman who feels a lump in her breast because a mammogram can't distinguish with certainty between a benign and a cancerous lump. The proper diagnostic test in Deliz's situation was an ultrasound.

Second, reassuring Deliz that a lump is "only calcification" is wrong for many reasons. Calcifications that can be seen on a mammogram don't produce a lump that anyone can feel because they are far too small (they are actually microscopic). Also, a cluster of microcalcifications is one of the classic mammographic appearances of breast cancer and not something to be dismissed.

Finally, any mass that is palpable (felt by the patient and the doctor) must be biopsied unless it is clearly a simple cyst confirmed by ultrasound examination.

Thankfully, Deliz did not simply accept her doctor's reassurance. Instead, she acted as her own advocate. Because of Deliz's actions, what could have been a disastrous delay of a year or more was "only" five months. Her persistence and her excellent response to preoperative chemotherapy mean that she has a very good chance of complete cure.

CHAPTER 5

Reaching A Correct Diagnosis Without Delay

"The best thing women can do for themselves is have regular mammograms."
—Christine Stewart

Despite all of the publicity regarding breast cancer, and the medical information available to doctors about how to correctly diagnose breast cancer, too many women have to wait too long to receive a correct diagnosis. This delay often leads to unnecessary suffering.

I recently reviewed the medical records of all the patients with breast cancer that I saw in my clinic at CTCA from March 2011 through February 2012. During that year, I saw 591 women with different stages and types of breast cancer. Many had been treated for years. In my review, I found that in ninety-five of these 591 women, their initial diagnosis was delayed at least six months, representing 16 percent, or nearly one in six women.

What's worse, the average delay between when the patient first felt a lump or abnormality to when she was correctly diagnosed was twelve months. As a result, by the time they came to CTCA, many of these patients had advanced disease that was much more difficult to treat effectively.

A serious medical condition like cancer should be diagnosed at the earliest possible moment and at the earliest possible stage. So what's causing these delays?

In sixty-six patients (11.3 percent of the total), the delay was caused by the patients themselves. They chose not to seek the advice of doctors even though each had felt a lump in her breast. Their lumps persisted and grew in size before these women finally sought medical help.

Twenty-three of the sixty-six patients who delayed seeking medical help tried to treat their cancers with a variety of natural means, such as herbs and diet. In those patients, the delay in receiving treatment was even longer, averaging eighteen months. Fourteen patients waited two years or even longer before seeing a doctor!

A total of twenty-seven women (4.5 percent of the total) went to see their doctors complaining of a lump and were incorrectly reassured that they "were fine," either based on the doctor's examination alone, or because the mammogram and sometimes an ultrasound examination didn't suggest cancer. No biopsies were taken.

Two women's diagnoses were delayed because they did not have prompt access to medical care: one was a victim of Hurricane Katrina, and the other didn't have health insurance.

Patient Delay: Facing Your Fear

What these numbers show is that in our patient population, **approximately one of every ten women who felt a cancerous lump in her breast suspected that she had cancer, and yet waited an entire year** on average before seeking appropriate medical care. This occurred here, in the United States—the country with arguably the best cancer care in the world and nearly constant media coverage about the importance of early detection of cancer.

Given all of the advances in early detection and treatment of breast cancer, these statistics should be a wakeup call to all of us. First, we have to understand *why* women are delaying seeking treatment. Second, doctors have to do a better job of communicating with their patients. And last, women have to educate themselves, take control of their medical care, and make appropriate treatment choices.

I believe the main reason women delay seeking treatment is fear. Some women deny the presence of cancer, others refuse treatment, and many are not appropriately educated about their cancer or given the opportunity to completely understand their condition and the options before them.

Fear frequently causes women to delay seeking medical help. Doctors must take the time to understand their patients and arm them with the best information possible about their condition so that patients can move beyond the fear of cancer and think rationally about their treatment options. Without strong communication and a trusting relationship, patients will often choose to delay or avoid treatment, sometimes with disastrous results.

According to the National Cancer Institute, 39,520 women died from breast cancer in 2011. Why? Many of these women were victims of biologically aggressive cancers, where the best of modern treatment is still not always successful. But others could have been saved if they had been diagnosed properly at the earliest possible time and received the best possible treatment.

It is very natural to be afraid if you feel a lump in your breast. But you can't allow fear to paralyze you. You have to seek medical attention. Because if the lump you feel is indeed cancer, then you need to start treatment right away. If it turns out not to be cancer, why subject yourself to months of needless worry? It is better to confront your fears and find out for sure using trusted diagnostic methods.

Driving this fear for many is a perception that a cancer diagnosis means inevitable suffering and certain death. But that's no longer true. **Most women diagnosed with breast cancer today can confidently expect to be completely cured.** And treatment is much, much easier than it was even twenty years ago.

The other primary fear is of the treatment itself, particularly fear of the side effects of chemotherapy. There have been tremendous advances in breast cancer treatment since I completed my training in the mid-1970s. Not only is treatment much more effective, but it is much more *tolerable* for the patient.

Consider these examples. Radical mastectomy, in which a woman loses the entire breast and underlying muscle, is rarely performed today. Most patients no longer require even a simple mastectomy and can be treated with breast-conserving surgery.

In my own field of medical oncology, there have been tremendous advances. Drug treatment is much more effective than it used to be. And it is much more tolerable. For example, the nausea and vomiting, which used to inevitably accompany chemotherapy can now be completely avoided.

All doctors who care for patients with breast cancer have the responsibility to fully educate them about exactly what their treatment plan will mean for them. Education and communication are key focuses of my practice; I spend as much time as necessary to ensure that each of my patients fully understands her condition and treatment options and can make an educated, thoughtful decision that is not driven by fear.

I also encourage patients facing their first breast cancer diagnosis to talk to a few patients who have been through the experience. At CTCA, many of our breast cancer survivors are happy to speak with new patients about their experience. Organizations can play a supportive role in helping women deal with the fear that inevitably accompanies breast cancer.

The bottom line is this: you can't allow fear to paralyze you. If you feel a lump in your breast, please see your doctor right away.

Doctor Errors Contribute to Delays in Treatment

In our study of 591 patients, twenty-seven women initially received an incorrect diagnosis from their doctors, delaying their treatment for six months or more. If this study is representative of the entire breast cancer population, it would suggest that up to ten thousand women are incorrectly diagnosed every year!

Doctor error causing delay in diagnosis is not a new phenomenon. In 2002, the Physician Insurers Association of America reported that delay in the diagnosis of breast cancer was the most common cause of malpractice lawsuits being filed. The study described more than one thousand cases in which the diagnosis of breast cancer was delayed. And as far back as 1993, the issue was discussed at a National Conference on Breast Cancer held in Boston where the major causes of delay in diagnosis were analyzed. The results are shown in the following table:

Major Reasons Doctors Fail to Diagnose Breast Cancer in a Timely Manner

1. Failure to order screening mammograms in asymptomatic woman (in other words, in women who felt fine)

2. Failure to have knowledge of or take appropriate action regarding an abnormal mammogram result

3. Failure to take patient symptoms seriously

4. Failure to verify patient complaint on physical examination

5. Failure to follow up on abnormal physical examination

6. Failure to refer patient to a breast specialist

7. Reliance on a false negative mammogram to exclude cancer in a patient with palpable mass

8. Failure to perform a biopsy when it was clearly needed

Most of the reasons for failing to promptly diagnose breast cancer shown in the table can be summarized in one sentence: the doctor failed to appreciate the significance of the patient's complaints, or relied on his or her examination or a negative mammogram to decide that the patient didn't in fact have cancer.

What can the patient do to prevent a delay in diagnosis?

If you feel a lump in your breast, you can't *force* your doctor to order a test or do a biopsy. But you can make sure that your doctor acts appropriately if your screening mammogram is reported as abnormal or (more commonly) if you feel something wrong with your breast.

So you, the patient, have to be a strong advocate for yourself. It isn't easy to say to a doctor, "I'm not satisfied with what you're telling me. I feel something in my breast, and I want it fully checked out by a specialist." Nor is it easy to request a second opinion.

But you have to be your own advocate. You have to ask questions. You have to be fully satisfied that your doctor has a sound scientific basis for whatever he or she is telling you, particularly if the doctor is not recommending a biopsy.

Take control of your health care and don't delay!

If you hear yourself or your doctor saying any of the following, then look out. You may be heading for serious trouble and absolutely should get a second opinion.

Below are some patient misconceptions about screening mammograms:

- When I had my last mammogram, it hurt a lot. I'm never doing that again!
- I'm not having a mammogram; my breasts feel fine. Why look for trouble?

- I'm really busy. I'll do the mammogram every couple of years.

Listed below are a few patient misconceptions about a breast lump:

- My mammogram was OK last year, so this lump can't be anything serious.
- The doctor told me my mammogram was fine, so I've got nothing to worry about.
- It's probably nothing.
- If I ignore it, it will go away.
- If I change my diet, it will go away (many variations).
- If I cut out sugar, meat, or coffee, it will go away (many variations).
- If I think positively, it will go away.
- If I boost my immune system, it will go away.
- It hurts, so I know it is not cancer.
- It doesn't hurt, so I know it is not cancer.

Misinformation from doctors about screening mammograms include the following:

- You don't need a mammogram. You're only forty.
- You don't need a mammogram. No one in your family had breast cancer.
- I don't believe in mammograms.

Below is misinformation given from doctors to women who feel a lump:

- You don't need a biopsy. It's just a milk duct.
- You don't need a biopsy. It's just a fibroid. (Women don't get fibroids in the breast. A fibroid is actually a benign muscle tumor of the uterus.)

- You don't need a biopsy. It's just a fibrocyst.
- You don't need a biopsy. I don't feel anything wrong.
- Women's breasts are always lumpy.
- You don't have cancer. There is no lump there.
- I know it is not cancer because you have no family history.
- You're too young for it to be cancer.
- It's just a cyst. It may get bigger before it goes away.
- You're pregnant, so your breasts always swell up.
- It's an infection. I'll give you antibiotics for ten days, and it'll clear up.
- I've got good news. The mammogram was normal.

Thus far, we have tried to give you a clear picture of how to reach a correct diagnosis without delay. Next, we will discuss what to do when a biopsy has been done and the doctor tells you that yes, the biopsy is positive for breast cancer.

What do you do now?

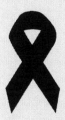

Early Diagnosis Leads to Better Treatment Results

WHEN TERRECE CRAWFORD WAS FORTY-FIVE YEARS OLD, she went for a routine checkup with her family doctor. She found an area of tenderness in her left breast. Terrece was (and still is) a healthy, young, single mother of two boys with no family history of breast cancer.

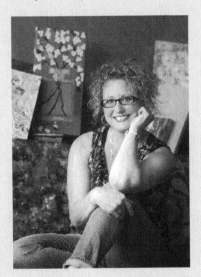

"It turns out that my cancer was growing very fast.
If I hadn't acted quickly, I might not be here today."
—Terrece Crawford

Terrece's doctor sent her for a mammogram, which showed no abnormality. (False negative mammograms are common in premenopausal women.) Despite the negative mammogram, her doctor also had ordered an ultrasound examination that showed a solid mass in the area of tenderness. A needle biopsy confirmed that this was a grade 2 ER-positive breast cancer.

"Early detection is so critical," Terrece says. "I insisted on having the ultrasound and biopsy on the same day because I wanted the information right away."

"My father was a doctor, and he died of cancer when I was only five years old," explained Terrece. "I had never imagined that I would partially understand his pain. Having breast cancer meant I could allow myself to grieve his loss in my life."

Terrece came to CTCA, where she was treated with surgery, radiation, chemotherapy, and estrogen-blocking hormone treatment. More than five years later, Terrece is completely cancer free, with an excellent prognosis for complete cure.

"It turns out that my cancer was growing very fast," she says. "If I hadn't acted quickly, I might not be here today. So my advice to women is: don't put it off, even for one day!"

Terrece is an artist, and during her cancer journey, she used art as therapy to help her maintain a positive attitude throughout treatment. "I even started teaching an art class at the hospital as a means of giving back and encouraging other patients/caregivers with an opportunity to express themselves."

"I would not have chosen to have breast cancer," Terrece concludes, "but I am thankful for the experiences I have had that have helped change my life to shape me into the woman I am now."

Doctor's Comments

The first sign of cancer in the breast is not always a lump. Breast cancer can also cause pain and tenderness in the breast.

Terrece has a tremendously positive attitude and is full of praise for us at CTCA, but the real hero is her family doctor who insisted on the ultrasound examination, despite the negative mammogram. Her story illustrates very clearly that a mammogram will not always show a breast cancer that is causing symptoms, particularly in young women.

The other heroine is Terrece herself. Breast cancer treatment is not easy, but she completed the entire treatment program with grace and courage.

CHAPTER 6

The Basic Principles of Breast Cancer Treatment (Part 1)

"Women are afraid of losing their hair? It's just hair! We shave it off of our legs every day! If you were diagnosed with diabetes, you'd get treatment for it. It's not a death sentence. It's just cancer."
—*Sandra Dillahunty*

If you have been diagnosed with breast cancer, don't panic. Most women diagnosed with breast cancer today are completely cured. Chances are very good that you will not die from breast cancer.

There are three very simple rules to follow to ensure that you receive the best possible treatment:

Rule One: You must understand the basic principles of breast cancer treatment.

Rule Two: You must choose doctors whom you trust to educate you and communicate freely and effectively with you.

Rule Three: You must commit to understanding and following your medical team's recommendations *completely*. Please resist the temptation to turn to the Internet or listen to the advice of family and friends. Their hearts are in the right place, but unless they are breast cancer specialists and know and understand all the details of your particular disease, the advice they provide could potentially be harmful.

The next two chapters are *not* intended to be a comprehensive description of *all* treatment options for the patient with breast cancer. Neither is it my intention to provide a *specific* treatment plan for any patient. Each individual patient needs a treatment plan that only her doctors can provide.

The goal here is to describe the basic principles of breast cancer treatment so that you will better understand what your doctors are recommending for you and the reasons behind those recommendations.

The most important fact about early breast cancer is this: **the best opportunity to be completely cured of breast cancer is when you are first diagnosed. The initial treatment plan is the one most likely to be curative.**

So what forms of treatment are available for the patient newly diagnosed with breast cancer? Broadly speaking, there are three main weapons doctors use: surgery, radiation, and drug treatment.

Cancer treatment has come a long way!

Historically and practically, surgery has always been the most important component of breast cancer treatment. In previous years, before core needle biopsy was available, surgery was also the most accurate process for diagnosing breast cancer (by surgical biopsy). Women would be put to sleep not knowing whether they had cancer. A surgical biopsy specimen would be examined while the patient was still under anesthesia (a "frozen section"), and if cancer were confirmed, the surgeon would immediately proceed to mastectomy. Patients would wake up after surgery, and immediately feel for their breast to determine whether it was still there.

I've been doing this work long enough that I remember seeing women who had been treated with the classic, radical mastectomy. The surgeon removed not only the entire breast, but also the underlying muscle all the way down to the chest wall. Women who had undergone radical mastectomy simply had skin covering their rib cages.

In addition, they often had severe lymphedema in their arms on the affected side, which was often three times bigger than the opposite arm. This was due to the extensive surgery of the axillary lymph nodes, often compounded by postoperative radiation.

Thankfully, we have moved very far from those days. Today, because of the availability of core needle biopsies, every woman can receive confirmation of the diagnosis in advance of surgery. We can learn a great deal of information about the stage of breast cancer and its biological type so that a detailed treatment plan can be developed. As a result, patients can (and should) have the opportunity to meet with all of their doctors and understand their treatment plan and the reasons for it *before* treatment ever begins.

Surgery of the Breast

There are basically two surgical operations available: a total mastectomy in which the whole breast is removed and a partial mastectomy (sometimes called lumpectomy) in which a part of the breast is removed. We often refer to partial mastectomy as breast-conserving surgery.

Sometimes a patient will be so afraid of cancer, she'll say, "I want the very best chance of cure, so take it off. In fact, take them both off." But the truth is that the cure rate for a lumpectomy is just as good as the cure rate for mastectomy. Removing the entire breast is unnecessary, provided that the surgical margins (the edges of the tissue that are removed) are free of cancer. If a patient chooses lumpectomy instead of total mastectomy, she will require some radiation to the remaining breast tissue.

Breast-conserving surgery is cosmetically, functionally, and psychologically more appropriate for most women than mastectomy.

There are, however, several special situations where mastectomy is necessary, and these are summarized below:

1. Multicentric cancer, where more than one cancer is present in different parts of the breast.

2. In cases with a very large tumor, usually four centimeters or bigger in diameter (approximately the size of a golf ball). Unless the patient has a very large breast, the amount of tissue to be removed would result in a cosmetically unacceptable result.*

(*This is not an absolute rule because we can often use drug treatment before surgery to reduce the size of the tumor in the breast. We call presurgical drug treatment *neo-adjuvant therapy*. The main advantage of this approach is to shrink the tumor so that the surgeon can remove a smaller amount of breast tissue than he or she would otherwise have to remove.)

3. Some women cannot receive postlumpectomy radiation because of a medical condition such as Lupus (radiation can cause severe tissue damage in these patients) or because they have already received radiation treatment to the breast or armpit area as treatment for an earlier breast cancer, DCIS, or other cancer, such as Hodgkin Disease. If the patient cannot receive radiation after surgery, lumpectomy is not an option, and mastectomy is the surgery of choice.

4. The final special situation relates to women who have a BRCA gene mutation. For these women, the risk of a second cancer is so high that removal of both breasts (bilateral mastectomy) may be the best option (more about BRCA later).

For those women who are treated with mastectomy, there are now several options available for breast reconstruction. A plastic or reconstructive surgeon is an important member of the breast cancer team, and I recommend that every woman contemplating mastectomy should meet with a reconstructive surgeon before mastectomy to discuss her options.

Your breast cancer team will recommend the most appropriate surgical treatment for you. To make that determination, the surgeon relies on information from the radiologist, who reads the imaging studies; the pathologist, who interprets the biopsy results and carefully checks all of the tissue removed to make sure all visible tumor has been removed; the radiation specialist, who works with the surgeon to plan radiation treatment either during or immediately after surgery; and the medical oncologist, who can predict how effective preoperative drug treatment may be in shrinking the tumor.

Most important of all, the surgeon must be guided by **you, the patient.** You have to clearly communicate your wishes and consider what is appropriate based on the realities of your specific medical condition.

Surgery of the Axillary Nodes

In addition to surgery on the breast, the lowest (sentinel) lymph node in the armpit (axilla) is also removed to check for spread of disease.

One of the major advances in breast cancer surgery in the past twenty years is the development of sentinel node sampling. This is a technique whereby only the lowest lymph node is removed. Prior to this, a much more extensive removal of lymph nodes (axillary dissection) was always performed, and in many cases, those nodes would contain no evidence of cancer. This more extensive surgery greatly increases the risk of long-term swelling of the arm (lymphedema).

Unless the lowest node in the armpit (the sentinel node) is shown to contain cancer, there is such a tiny risk of cancer in the other nodes that surgeons have now largely abandoned routine axillary dissection in favor of sentinel node sampling. A recent large study has challenged the need for axillary dissection even if the sentinel node is involved. So this is a decision that every patient must discuss fully with her surgeon before she has surgery.

The modern approach is to *do less treatment but achieve the same result, namely total cure.* In nearly all cases, treatment is not finished with surgery. There is also a need for additional local treatment in the form of radiation therapy and systemic drug treatment (adjuvant therapy).

Radiation

Radiation is a form of local treatment. Most of us are familiar with medical X-rays. When patients are exposed to the same type of X-rays but in a much higher dose and for a longer time, those X-rays will damage the exposed tissue and cells. We make use of this phenomenon by using high energy X-rays to kill cancer cells (radiation therapy).

In the patient with breast cancer, radiation therapy is used to kill any microscopic (undetectable) cancer cells, which may remain in the breast, chest wall, or nodal areas (armpit and just above the collarbone) after surgery is completed. We use radiation to further increase the probability of preventing cancer recurrence in these areas.

In the patient who has chosen breast-conserving surgery (lumpectomy rather than mastectomy), we radiate either the tumor bed, meaning the area of the breast immediately surrounding where the tumor was, or the entire breast tissue after surgery.

In patients at higher-than-average risk because of a larger tumor in the breast, and/or lymph nodes involved, we include the nodal areas in the radiation field.

Not every patient requires radiation. If a woman elects to have a simple mastectomy and has cancer-free sentinel nodes, she will in all likelihood not require radiation. On occasion, when treating a woman with a larger tumor or multiple nodes involved, we will recommend radiation, even when the patient has had a total mastectomy because of a higher risk of the disease recurring in the future.

There are now a variety of newer radiation techniques in which the doctor can radiate all or only part of the breast tissue remaining after surgery. It is now even possible for some patients to complete their radiation treatment during surgery through a process known as intraoperative radiation treatment (IORT). This major advance means that some patients can now be treated for one day only (during surgery) rather than have weeks of postoperative radiation treatment. It must be stressed that this new approach is not for every patient, but depends on the type of breast cancer, the geometry of the individual patient's breast, and the technology available at the specific hospital.

Side Effects of Radiation Therapy

For most patients with early breast cancer, radiation will produce short-term burning of the skin of the irradiated area (like a bad sunburn). Such local reactions are almost always completely reversible with time, and rarely produce long-term problems for the patient.

Of greater concern are more severe side effects that can occur, often many years after treatment. The most important of these is a rare cancer *caused by* radiation called **angiosarcoma.** Some patients develop angiosarcoma following radiation treatment for breast cancer.

The risk of radiation-induced cancer has to be seen in context, however. In a Swedish study of nearly fourteen thousand patients with breast cancer treated with radiation, less than one in one thousand patients developed a sarcoma due to that radiation. We have to balance this very small number of cancers against the fact that radiation after breast cancer surgery reduces the risk of local recurrence of the cancer in the breast by 80 percent.

Systemic Drug Treatment

Surgery and radiation are local treatments aimed at a particular part of the body. Systemic drug treatment is designed to kill cancer cells present anywhere in the body. When a patient receives drug treatment (either through injections or pills), the drugs are absorbed into the bloodstream and carried throughout the body. Wherever the blood carries the drug, it will come into contact with cancer cells and hopefully kill them.

So the advantage of drug treatment over local treatment is that it provides the potential for killing cancer cells wherever they are in the body. Drug treatment for breast cancer includes chemotherapy, hormone treatments, and drugs such as trastuzumab, which attack the specific cellular targets we described earlier (HER2neu).

Almost every patient diagnosed with invasive breast cancer will require some form of drug treatment. A consultation with a medical oncologist—the care provider specially trained in cancer medicine and the safe use of chemotherapy and the other drugs—is an essential part of the treatment plan of every patient with breast cancer.

Chemotherapy

Medical oncologists treat cancer with cytotoxic drugs that kill living cells, commonly known as *chemotherapy*. Chemotherapy has been used for more than fifty years to treat patients with cancer with varying degrees of success. Among the common cancers that we treat, breast cancer is among the most sensitive to chemotherapy. There are a large number of chemotherapy drugs that have shown the ability to kill breast cancer cells.

Some Chemotherapy Drugs Active Against Breast Cancer

Paclitaxel protein-bound	Gemcitabine
Doxorubicin	Ixabepilone
Carboplatin	Vinorelbine
Cyclophosphamide	Paclitaxel
Doxorubicin liposomal	Docetaxel
Eribulin mesylate	Capecitabine

Chemotherapy is used to control advanced disease, and also to prevent recurrence (and therefore increase overall cure rate) when given to patients after surgery for early stage breast cancer. We call this *adjuvant therapy*.

Possible Side Effects of Chemotherapy

Our ability to prevent or minimize the side effects of chemotherapy has greatly improved over the past ten years, and overall the *benefits* of chemotherapy far outweigh the *risks*.

Many people are very afraid of chemotherapy and often have an exaggerated idea of the side effects (toxicity) of this form of cancer treatment. When doctors talk about the risks of any treatment, they are referring to unwanted and negative effects of treatment that are different from the desired effect. Obviously, the desired effect we always want is the disappearance of or at least shrinkage of the cancerous tumor. But other effects also may occur, and we call these *side effects*.

It is certainly true that we see more side effects from the drugs we use to treat patients with cancer when compared with drugs used for patients being treated for other chronic diseases like diabetes, rheumatoid arthritis, or high blood pressure (hypertension).

But we have to remember that cancer represents a very fundamental change in the structure of cells and tissues, and breast cancer is a potentially lethal disease. **So cancer doctors *have to* use very powerful drugs that unfortunately can cause severe side effects in some patients.**

While we mustn't overestimate these side effects, it is important that patients fully understand what the side effects might be before they start chemotherapy:

- Older chemotherapy was often associated with severe side effects. As a result, chemotherapy developed a very bad reputation, and most patients are very apprehensive when they are told that they need chemotherapy. The fact is we are much better today at controlling and preventing side effects than we were in the past.
- Many years ago, many patients treated with chemotherapy experienced severe vomiting soon after receiving their treatment. We now have modern drugs that act directly on the vomiting center

of the brain, and give several of these drugs to patients immediately before they receive chemotherapy. **As a result, severe nausea and vomiting after chemotherapy are a thing of the past. I tell all my patients the following: if you throw up as a result of chemo, it means I'm not doing my job properly.**

- The side effects that cannot be avoided are hair loss, tiredness, and the suspension of menstruation. With most chemotherapy drugs, the hair loss is complete and usually occurs within a few weeks of starting treatment, but it is temporary. Within six months, your hair will start growing back. For those who are only receiving short-term treatment in the adjuvant setting, your hair should completely grow back within a year.

- Regarding tiredness, the fatigue is very real, and there is no magic pill that will help. You'll feel very tired for a few days after the chemo and will have to rest. Listen to your body. If you're tired, just rest. This is when your family can really help. Your number one priority must be YOU.

- The third side effect that can't be avoided is a cessation of menstruation in premenopausal women.

I want to mention three other side effects that merit special attention. These include lowering of the levels of white blood cells and platelets in the blood; damage to nerves; and finally, what is often referred to as "chemo brain."

Lowering of White Blood Cells and Platelets

Chemotherapy is designed to kill cancer cells that are actively growing (reproducing). We are constantly making new blood cells in our bone marrow, so most chemotherapy drugs will inevitably also kill some healthy bone marrow and result in a temporary lowering of the level of circulating blood cells. This is why patients being treated with chemotherapy must have their blood counts checked regularly.

Of particular concern is the increased risk for infection caused by fewer white blood cells and reduced platelet count that can be associated with increased risk of bleeding. When bleeding occurs, it is usually not serious (skin bruises or a nose bleed), but it is certainly something that your doctor should know.

The good news is that new medications are now available to minimize damage to the bone marrow.

Damage to Nerve Tissue (Neuropathy)

Many of the chemotherapy drugs that are most active against breast cancer have the potential for causing damage to nerve tissue, particularly the long nerves in the arms and legs. We call this condition Peripheral Neuropathy, and it is usually recognized by the patient as tingling, pins and needles, and numbness of her fingers and toes.

Peripheral Neuropathy rarely occurs with the first chemotherapy treatment and is more common when treatment extends over several months or longer. The naturopathic providers on our Breast Cancer Team can often effectively prevent or treat neuropathy with a combination of B vitamins, essential fatty acids and/or L-glutamine. If these are not wholly effective, there are prescription drugs that can be used to provide real benefit.

Chemo Brain

Chemo brain is the name given to the mental fog and memory issues that some patients describe while they are being treated with chemotherapy. Some patients report that these difficulties may persist for years after chemotherapy is completed.

A recent study has suggested that women treated with chemotherapy twenty years earlier perform less well on memory tests and tests of thinking and hand movement ("cognitive skills") when compared with women who never received chemotherapy.

It may be difficult to identify subtle loss of cognitive function, but I have little doubt that chemotherapy can affect some women adversely in this regard. As breast cancer treatment becomes more successful and more women are being cured, it is likely that we will see more of this phenomenon in long-term survivors. It is important not to exaggerate this effect. The recent study referenced estimated the magnitude of the decline in mental function to the equivalent of six years of aging.

Serious brain damage, such as dementia or Alzheimer's Disease, has never been reported from chemotherapy treatment, and it appears that chemo brain is not a major problem for most women.

This is another area where our naturopathic providers, registered dieticians, and mind-body specialists make a major contribution. They have found that a healthy diet that includes supplements of B vitamins and folic acid may be beneficial in reducing the risk of chemo brain.

There are many other side effects that patients receiving chemotherapy may experience. I always emphasize that many of the side effects listed are *possible*, but not definite. In general terms, if chemotherapy is given carefully and within accepted dosage guidelines, side effects are manageable, and the disadvantages of treatment are greatly outweighed by the benefits (cure or at least remission from cancer).

Hormone Therapy

Female sex hormones, particularly estrogen, stimulate the growth of normal breast cells by binding to the cell membrane. This binding requires the presence of a specific, estrogen-binding protein called the *estrogen receptor* (ER).

Like a key fitting into a lock, the binding of estrogen and ER switches the cell "on" and causes it to divide, resulting in the growth of breast tissue. But this process also causes breast cancer cells to grow.

In 1888, a brilliant surgeon by the name of William Beatson in Glasgow, Scotland, was the first to recognize that he could control the ravages of advanced breast cancer in young women by removing their ovaries, and therefore cutting off the production of estrogen. Beatson reasoned correctly that denying the cancer the stimulation of estrogen produced by the ovaries would cause the cancer to die.

Seventy years later another brilliant doctor named Charles Huggins at the University of Chicago essentially repeated the same experiment by removing the testes (the source of testosterone) in men with advanced prostate cancer. (Huggins was eventually awarded the Nobel Prize for this discovery.)

Although generally referred to as *hormone therapy* for breast cancer, it is actually antihormone or hormone-blocking treatment, designed either to reduce the body's levels of estrogen to an absolute minimum or to prevent the estrogen in the body from stimulating the growth of any remaining breast cancer cells.*

*Hormone therapy should not be confused with Hormone Replacement Therapy (HRT), the practice of giving estrogen to women to relieve or prevent symptoms of menopause, which are related to a lack of estrogen. The combination of estrogen and progesterone significantly increases a woman's risk for developing breast cancer, and it is not a practice that I recommend. I also strongly oppose giving supplemental estrogens to women who have been diagnosed and treated for breast cancer, except in special circumstances, which are very rare, and only under the closest of medical supervision.

So why is estrogen-blocking therapy so important for the treatment of the patient with breast cancer, and not, for example, helpful for patients with other common cancers like bowel or lung cancer?

The simple answer is **hormone receptors**. As we described in Chapter 2, many breast cancer cells contain the estrogen receptor, while bowel and lung cancer cells do not. It's the presence of ER, which makes breast cancer cells highly sensitive to hormone therapy.

If your doctor tells you that your breast cancer is ER-positive (estrogen-receptor positive), you can be pretty sure that part of your treatment will be a pill or other medical procedure designed to either interfere with your ability to produce estrogen, or block the effect of estrogen on your cancer cells.

The following are ways that doctors can inhibit stimulation of the breast cancer cell by estrogen, including a few general points about hormone treatment:

- First, hormone therapy is used to treat patients with advanced breast cancer. It is also used as adjuvant therapy in addition to surgery in patients with early stage breast cancer. In that context, it is very effective in reducing the risk of recurrent disease and therefore increasing overall cure rates.
- Second, hormone therapy is not indicated to treat patients with ER-negative (hormone insensitive) breast cancer.
- Third, when treating patients with advanced disease, shrinkage of tumors tends to occur more slowly with hormone therapy than with chemotherapy. However, hormone-induced remissions do tend to persist longer, often for years. Doctors say that hormone-induced responses are more *durable*.
- Finally, when compared with chemotherapy, hormone treatment side effects are usually much less significant than with chemotherapy. But, all hormone treatments designed to reduce or otherwise interfere with a woman's estrogen levels may produce undesirable side effects that can interfere with a patient's quality of life. These may include weight gain, hot flashes, vaginal dryness that often causes painful intercourse, and reduced libido (sex drive).
- Undesirable side effects may encourage patients to refuse hormone treatment or stop their treatment early, which can negatively affect their outcomes. In Chapter 12, we will discuss the critical importance of patients completing the treatment plan that their doctors have recommended.

Hormone-Blocking Therapy for the Patient with Breast Cancer

Premenopausal Women:

- Surgical removal of ovaries
- Drugs that stop the ovary from producing estrogen (LH-RH agonists)
- Tamoxifen
- Fulvestrant

Postmenopausal Women:

- Aromatase Inhibitors
- Fulvestrant
- Everolimus

- A recent major study in Europe has shown that continued use of hormone-blocking treatment for ten years after surgery for early state breast cancer results in significantly fewer lapses or recurrences of the disease. It is likely that this will become the standard practice here in the United States.

Notes about Tamoxifen

Tamoxifen has been used to treat women with breast cancer for more than forty years. Tamoxifen is a very effective drug and has helped hundreds of thousands of women with breast cancer. But, like every other drug, there are possible side effects associated with tamoxifen:

- About 2 percent of patients treated with tamoxifen will develop a blood clot in the veins of the leg, which may on occasion travel to the lung (a serious condition called pulmonary embolism).
- Tamoxifen increases the risk of two types of cancer of the uterus. The risk of cancer of the lining of the uterus (endometrium) is approximately two cases per thousand women taking tamoxifen (compared with one case per thousand in women not on tamoxifen). This is usually a low-grade cancer treated by hysterectomy.
- Much less common (less than one case per thousand) and more serious is uterine sarcoma, a cancer of the muscle of the uterine wall; incidence is slightly increased by tamoxifen use.

Many women are afraid to take tamoxifen because of its possible side effects. It is important to emphasize that serious side effects such as blood clots and cancer are, in fact, very uncommon. The vast majority of women treated with tamoxifen do not experience serious toxicity.

Whenever tamoxifen or any other treatment is considered, the patient with breast cancer and her doctor have to weigh the risks of side effects against the benefits of long-term control (or cure) of her cancer.

Aromatase Inhibitors

In premenopausal women, most estrogen is produced in the ovaries. Estrogen levels are much lower after menopause, when the ovaries are no longer functioning. While estrogen levels are much lower in postmenopausal women, they are not zero. Estrogen is still produced in muscle tissue, body fat, and a small gland located just above the kidneys called the adrenal gland. Estrogen is produced in these sites by an enzyme called *Aromatase*, and can be inhibited by a class of drugs called *aromatase inhibitors*.

Even low levels of estrogen can stimulate the growth of ER-positive breast cancer cells, and aromatase inhibitors have been shown to be a very effective form of treatment for ER-positive (hormone-sensitive) breast cancer in postmenopausal women. Aromatase inhibitors are used to treat women with advanced breast cancer and also after surgery to prevent recurrence, much like tamoxifen is used in premenopausal women.

Aromatase inhibitors are simple pills taken once a day. Because they lower estrogen levels and produce what I call a "super menopause," they can cause vaginal dryness, reduced libido (sex drive), worsening of hot flashes, and can slightly increase the long-term risk of bone thinning (osteoporosis). They can also cause weight gain and a curious arthritis-like joint pain.

Many of the sexual side effects of aromatase inhibitors could be avoided by prescribing estrogen, and there are some doctors who have recommended the use of low dose estrogen cream applied directly to the vagina to relieve the symptoms of atrophic vaginitis (dryness and discomfort).

There is, however, evidence that estrogen applied to the vagina is absorbed, and measurable levels of estrogen can be detected in the blood after vaginal administration.

This is not surprising when you think that many drugs are administered as skin patches (think of pain meds, nicotine patches, nitro patches for angina, and estrogen!).

The risk of giving vaginal estrogen cream to breast cancer patients is that the estrogen might stimulate the growth of any estrogen sensitive cancer cells that remain in the body, resulting in relapse of the cancer.

I do not recommend that any woman with a history of breast cancer should ever be prescribed an estrogen-containing drug, including vaginal estrogen cream.

There is good news, however, for women who experience sexual side effects from breast cancer treatment. The FDA recently approved Ospemifine, a nonestrogen pill, for the treatment of painful intercourse. Ospemifine reverses the physical changes in the vagina caused by lack of estrogen. And, paroxetine, widely used to treat depression, is the only nonhormonal pill approved by the FDA to treat hot flashes.

Unlike tamoxifen, aromatase inhibitors do not cause serious side effects, such as an increased risk of blood clots or uterine cancer. In general, their side effects are relatively mild and manageable and are greatly outweighed by the benefits of treatment. We have found that some patients find great benefit from working with naturopathic providers to minimize the side effects of aromatase inhibitors.

Resistance to Hormone Treatment

One of the problems with drug treatment of breast cancer is the development of *drug resistance*. After a period of time, a drug (chemotherapy or hormone) that has been effective in controlling the disease loses its effectiveness, and the cancer starts to grow again despite continued treatment with the same drug. Drug resistance occurs because the cancer apparently is smart enough to undergo certain mutations or changes in its chemistry that are favorable to its growth.

In the past, when a cancer developed resistance to a specific drug or class of drugs, we would have to stop using that drug, but a recent development offers a major new approach to the problem.

A recent study, called the BOLERO-2 trial, has shown that a drug called everolimus could counteract acquired resistance to hormone therapy in postmenopausal women with hormone receptor-positive metastatic breast cancer.

The results of this study are very exciting, as they provide an entirely new way that women with ER-positive breast cancer may continue to benefit from hormone treatment. Based on those results, the FDA approved everolimus in combination with an aromatose inhibitor in July 2012.

This is an example of how recent advances in our understanding of the biology of breast cancer are providing real improvements in treatment for thousands of women.

Trastuzumab and HER2neu

The target for hormone blockers is the estrogen receptor (ER). The goal is to either prevent estrogen from binding to the receptor by blocking it with tamoxifen, or to reduce the body's production of estrogen. However it is done, the goal is to switch off the estrogen pathway that stimulates the growth of ER-positive breast cancer cells. There are other cellular targets in some breast cancers, the most important of which is HER2neu.

In 1998, a drug called trastuzumab first became available to treat women with HER2neu-positive breast cancer. Trastuzumab is a protein (an antibody), which specifically binds to and inactivates the HER2neu receptor. As a result, the HER2neu protein is inactivated and can't promote tumor cell growth.

Although the cellular targets are different, both tamoxifen and trastuzumab are examples of modern medical oncology where the emphasis has moved from cytotoxic chemotherapy (which to some extent kills *all* cells) to more specific therapy that targets specific proteins that have been identified in cancer cells as opposed to healthy cells.

Targeted therapies are much more specific and therefore more effective and less toxic to healthy cells, so there are often less side effects than with chemotherapy.

Trastuzumab has been so successful in treating patients with advanced or recurrent HER2neu-positive breast cancer that it is now used in the *adjuvant* setting to prevent tumor recurrences in patients with early stage disease.

Before leaving the subject of HER2neu-positive breast cancer, it is important to mention that trastuzumab is only the first of what promises to be a large number of treatments directed against HER2neu and the cellular processes that it mediates.

There are several other drugs, including lapatinib, neratinib, pertuzumab, and ado-trastuzumab emtansine that also show significant activity against HER2neu-positive disease.

In summary, the three main forms of treatment for breast cancer are surgery, radiation, and drug treatment. Each treatment is prescribed and supervised by a different kind of cancer specialist. The next chapter details how each of these forms of treatment is used to treat patients with different stages of breast cancer.

CHAPTER 7

The Basic Principles of Breast Cancer Treatment (Part 2)

"Having cancer is almost like being turned wrong-side-out, given a few good shakes, and then put right-side-out again, all fresh and clean. Cancer doesn't have to be horrible. You can allow it to change your life in a positive way."
—Iva "Marie" Botchie

The vast majority of patients with breast cancer are diagnosed with early stage breast cancer. In fact, less than one in twenty breast patients with cancer are first diagnosed with Stage IV disease. **Women need to know that early stage breast cancer is a very curable disease!**

This chapter outlines broad principles of treatment based on stage of disease at the time of first diagnosis. We will discuss treatment of patients with different stages of breast cancer:

Stage 0: Patients with preinvasive breast cancer (DCIS)

Stages I and II: Patients with early stage invasive breast cancer

Stage III: Patients with locally advanced breast cancer

Stage IV: Patients with distant metastases

Stage O: Preinvasive Disease (Ductal Carcinoma in Situ, or DCIS)

DCIS is *not* invasive breast cancer. While the cells seen in a biopsy are cancer cells with all of the characteristics of cancer cells, they have not yet invaded out of the breast duct. So DCIS is noninvasive, or more accurately, *preinvasive* cancer.

It is likely that all invasive cancer starts out as preinvasive cancer. So we treat DCIS for one important reason: to prevent the subsequent development of invasive breast cancer.

The basic principle of treatment for the patient with DCIS is to simply remove or destroy all traces of DCIS in the breast. Generally, treatment involves surgically removing the affected area, and then administering radiation to some or all of the remainder of the breast. Radiation therapy is critical to ensuring that any abnormal cells left behind after surgery are destroyed and cannot cause a recurrence of DCIS or develop into invasive cancer in the future.

Sometimes local surgery of the affected area is not enough to cure DCIS. The ducts affected by DCIS can extend widely throughout the breast. (Refer to the diagram on page 17, showing how the ducts extend throughout the breast like the roots of a plant.) When DCIS has extended through a large part of the ductal system, there is only one form of treatment that is 100 percent effective: a simple mastectomy, in which the surgeon removes the entire breast. When mastectomy is used to treat DCIS, there is no need for radiation. Using a mastectomy to treat DCIS eliminates the need for radiation.

DCIS is usually diagnosed through a mammogram because of the presence of irregular, so-called pleomorphic calcifications. Mammograms are also effective at showing how extensive the abnormal calcifications may be. After removal, a pathologist will check the removed tissue and inform the surgeon that all surgical margins are clear of DCIS.

If you have DCIS, the three most important doctors involved in your care are the radiologist, surgeon, and pathologist working closely together.

Drug Treatment for DCIS

There is absolutely no place for chemotherapy in the treatment of DCIS. But what about hormone-blocking (antiestrogen) therapy?

Tamoxifen is approved for the *prevention* of breast cancer in women at higher than average risk for developing the disease. So does it make sense to take tamoxifen after surgery for DCIS?

There are somewhat conflicting results from two large studies in which tamoxifen was given after definitive local treatment for DCIS. One study was done in the United States, and the other was done in Europe. The studies concluded that there appears to be no improvement in overall survival rates with the use of tamoxifen (not surprising when you remember that DCIS is almost 100 percent curable with local treatment alone). But there was a small but statistically significant reduction in the incidence of future breast cancer development in those women who were given tamoxifen, at least in the US study.

So in the United States, doctors frequently recommend five years of hormone-blocking therapy, using either tamoxifen or an aromatase inhibitor, depending on whether the patient is still menstruating.

And finally, every woman treated for DCIS needs to have a mammogram every year for the rest of her life.

Stages I and II: Early Stage Disease

Most women with early breast cancer (Stage I and Stage II) can expect to be completely cured of their disease. By cure we mean complete eradication of the disease, without a recurrence, and with the same life expectancy as any other woman of similar age.

There are two basic principles of treatment for the patient with early breast cancer. One is focused on local treatment, which is accomplished by totally removing or destroying all traces of the cancer in the breast and any involved lymph nodes: the armpit (axilla) and the area above the collarbone (supra-clavicular area). Local treatment comprises surgery, often combined with some radiation.

The second principle of treatment is the use of some form of drug treatment to kill any cancer cells that may have already spread from the local area of the breast and axillary nodes to more distant sites. In contrast with local treatment, drug treatment is systemic, meaning it is designed to kill cancer cells that may have spread anywhere in the body.

Because drug treatment is given *in addition* to local treatment, you'll often hear this referred to as *adjuvant therapy*. The purpose of adjuvant therapy is to increase the probability of total cure by preventing the future development of secondary tumors (metastases).

In some patients with apparently early breast cancer, some cancer cells may already be present in distant sites, even though we can't see them or identify their presence with even the most sophisticated blood tests, CAT scan, or MRI scan. Left untreated, they will grow silently for years until they reach a critical mass and cause symptoms that lead to their discovery. That is referred to as a relapse, or recurrence, of the cancer.

History of Adjuvant Therapy

Up until 1970 or so, the standard treatment for women with breast cancer was mastectomy, followed by radiation therapy to the chest wall (where the breast was removed) and the armpit. And for many thousands of women, this treatment plan was perfectly adequate. The cancer never recurred, and they were cured. But for many other women, the cancer came back, either in the general area of the chest wall or armpit, or at more distant sites, such as bone, liver, or lung. At that time, such recurrent breast cancer was incurable.

Then in the 1970s, chemotherapy drugs were discovered to be effective at killing breast cancer cells. When patients with advanced breast cancer were treated with chemotherapy drugs, a small but significant percentage of patients showed obvious tumor shrinkage. Based on this, some very smart doctors reasoned that giving chemotherapy to patients with breast cancer would help to prevent recurrence and therefore increase the cure rate. This theory was tested by giving one half of the patients chemotherapy and comparing the results with a group of patients who did not receive chemotherapy after surgery (the control group). Following these early studies, additional research has allowed us to refine and modify our treatment recommendations.

Over the past forty years, clinical research studies have been conducted in thousands of women with early breast cancer. These studies have consistently shown that women who receive adjuvant treatment have significantly lower rates of recurrent cancer and therefore higher cure rates than women who don't receive such treatment. It is now recommended in all but the most favorable cases of invasive breast cancer.

Why Adjuvant Therapy Is Critical

When patients are given adjuvant therapy (chemotherapy and/or hormone therapy), we don't *know* for sure that she still has cancer in her body. We give the treatment because of the *possibility* or *probability* that there are still some cancer cells remaining after local treatment has been completed. And the concern is that unless these cells are killed, they will cause a recurrence of the cancer in the future. The probability of future recurrence is estimated based on the presence of one or more of the risk factors (discussed in Chapter 2).

It is sometimes difficult for patients to fully accept the need for and importance of adjuvant therapy because at the time they are being treated, there is no evidence of cancer, and they can't see an immediate benefit from the treatment. **However, it is critically important that patients understand its importance, trust the medical team's advice, and complete the recommended treatment program.** This is particularly true for patients with ER-positive breast cancer who must complete *years* of adjuvant, hormone-blocking treatment and are sometime reluctant to do so.

It should be emphasized that not all women require adjuvant chemotherapy. The medical oncologist on your treatment team will determine if you need adjuvant therapy and what specific treatment is most appropriate for you. The decision whether to be treated with adjuvant chemotherapy is based on an evaluation of your risk of future recurrence of disease (discussed in Chapter 2). **But every woman diagnosed with invasive breast cancer should have a consultation with a medical oncologist to discuss the need for adjuvant therapy.**

Types of Adjuvant Therapy

Adjuvant therapy may take the form of chemotherapy, hormone therapy or trastuzumab, or a combination of these drugs, depending on whether the tumor is positive for estrogen receptor (ER), or HER2neu. This is where the modern biological typing of the cancer we discussed in Chapter 2 is absolutely critical in ensuring that every woman gets the drug treatment tailored to her specific type of cancer.

Chemotherapy is usually given for approximately four to six months. For women with ER-positive (estrogen sensitive) early breast cancer, estrogen-blocking drugs ("endocrine treatment") have traditionally been prescribed for a period of five years after surgery as additional (adjuvant) treatment to prevent recurrence of disease. Recent studies have shown a clear benefit in terms of reduced risk of cancer recurrence when tamoxifen treatment was continued for a period of ten years after initial surgery.

If these results are confirmed in studies of other endocrine treatment, it is likely that at least ten years of adjuvant endocrine treatment will become the new norm. For a patient with HER2neu-positive cancer, it is currently recommended that she receive one year of trastuzumab treatment in addition to chemotherapy.

There is a very informative website developed for doctors and patients called Adjuvant! Online that clearly shows how effective drug treatment (chemotherapy and hormone-blocking) can be in reducing the risk of future relapse of disease when used after surgery as adjuvant therapy in patients with early breast cancer. The relevant details of every case of breast cancer can be entered into the program. The following is an example that shows the benefit of chemotherapy and hormone therapy derived from the Adjuvant Online! website:

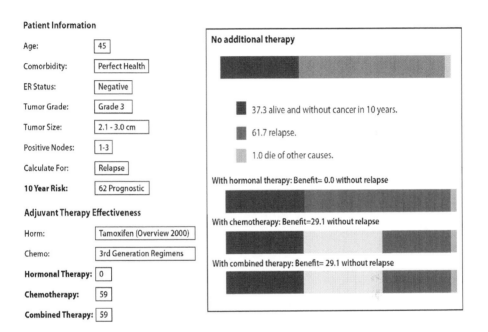

Patient Information

Age:	45
Comorbidity:	Perfect Health
ER Status:	Negative
Tumor Grade:	Grade 3
Tumor Size:	2.1 - 3.0 cm
Positive Nodes:	1-3
Calculate For:	Relapse
10 Year Risk:	62 Prognostic

Adjuvant Therapy Effectiveness

Horm:	Tamoxifen (Overview 2000)
Chemo:	3rd Generation Regimens
Hormonal Therapy:	0
Chemotherapy:	59
Combined Therapy:	59

No additional therapy

- 37.3 alive and without cancer in 10 years.
- 61.7 relapse.
- 1.0 die of other causes.

With hormonal therapy: Benefit= 0.0 without relapse

With chemotherapy: Benefit=29.1 without relapse

With combined therapy: Benefit= 29.1 without relapse

This hypothetical example shows a forty-five-year-old, premenopausal woman in perfect health who recently had surgical removal of a 2.5-centimeter, high-grade tumor (grade 3), ER-negative with two lymph nodes containing cancer. This is a common situation in which chemotherapy is recommended.

What the Adjuvant Online! computer model shows is the following: Imagine one hundred patients just like her, and all refused drug treatment after surgery and radiation. Without any drug treatment, approximately sixty-one out of one hundred women would have a recurrence of cancer within ten years, and almost all would eventually die from breast cancer.

By taking the recommended chemotherapy treatment (for approximately six months), twenty-nine of the sixty-one women would avoid a relapse of their disease and remain cancer free. As the tumor was ER negative, hormone treatment is not effective and is not recommended.

It is clear from this example that adjuvant therapy offers significant benefit to patients with early stage breast cancer. In my experience, patients find this computer program a very useful educational tool in helping them to understand the real and definite benefits of adjuvant treatment.

Neo-Adjuvant Therapy

Neo-adjuvant therapy refers to the concept of giving drug treatment (usually chemotherapy but sometimes hormone treatment) *before* surgery. Giving chemotherapy before surgery (neo-adjuvant therapy) is just as likely to increase overall cure rate as conventional adjuvant therapy (given after surgery). Many studies have shown that either approach is equally effective.

The main advantage of giving drug treatment before surgery is that, in many cases, we are able to shrink the cancer so much that the surgeon can remove much less healthy breast tissue. In many cases, women who would otherwise require a mastectomy can be successfully treated with breast-conserving surgery ("lumpectomy") following preoperative drug treatment.

Before we leave the subject of early breast cancer, I want to emphasize again that by using all three forms of treatment available (surgery, radiation, and drug treatment), **most women with early stage breast cancer can confidently expect to be completely cured of their disease.**

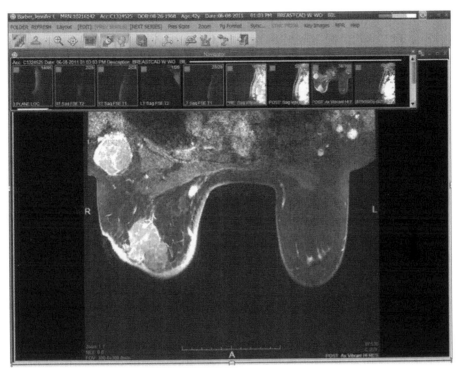

MRI of the breasts of patient Jennifer Barber (discussed in the introduction) at her first evaluation at CTCA shows a massive tumor in the right breast with very large metastasis in the right axillary lymph node. Note also the thickening of the skin of the right breast. Without preoperative drug treatment, Jennifer would have undoubtedly required mastectomy.

Stage III: Locally Advanced Disease

Stage III disease is defined as breast cancer in which the primary tumor in the breast is larger than five centimeters (about two inches) in greatest diameter, or there is heavy involvement of the axillary (armpit) lymph nodes, which are enlarged and often matted together. The three basic treatments recommended for Stage III breast cancer are the same as earlier stage disease, namely surgery, radiation, and drug treatment. The difference between treatment of patients with

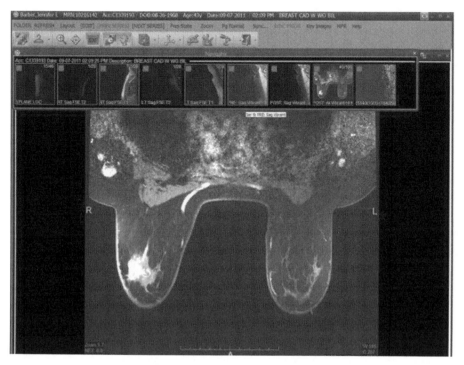

MRI of Jennifer Barber's breasts following four treatments with preoperative (neo-adjuvant) chemotherapy. There has been significant shrinkage of the mass in the breast and axilla. Note also the normal appearance of the skin of the right breast. At the time of surgery, there was no residual cancer in the breast or axilla. The abnormality seen on the MRI simply represents scar tissue. Jennifer was able to avoid mastectomy, and her prognosis for cure is excellent.

Stages I, II, or III cancers is in the *sequencing, intensity,* and *duration* of treatment.

With Stage III disease, there is no one hard and fast rule for treatment. The treatment plan for a patient with Stage III disease is highly individualized, and the initial plan may well be modified as doctors observe the response of the tumor in the breast and node to therapy. Most treatment plans for patients with Stage III disease include neo-adjuvant treatment before surgery.

With modern combined treatment plans using a combination of chemotherapy, surgery, and radiation, the outlook for many patients with Stage III disease is greatly improved, and long-term control of the disease (for years) is often achieved.

Stage IV: Distant Metastatic Disease

Less than 5 percent of women have Stage IV breast cancer when first diagnosed. In these patients, the symptoms of disease are due to secondary tumors that have developed because of the spread of cancer from an unrecognized (or sometimes ignored) cancer in the breast. Since these secondary tumors are called metastases, the patient is described as having *metastatic breast cancer*.

Most commonly, the patient's symptoms are due to metastatic spread of the cancer into bone, chest, or the abdominal cavity. Bone tumors commonly cause pain, usually in the back. Occasionally the first sign of cancer in bone is the development of a fracture, usually in a weight-bearing bone, such as the hip or thigh bone. These are called *pathologic* fractures and differ from fractures that occur in healthy bone following an injury, since they may occur with little or no trauma.

Metastatic breast cancer may be identified because the patient develops a cough or shortness of breath due to disease in the chest or abdominal pain or other signs of cancer in the abdomen. This is particularly likely to occur with lobular cancer of the breast (discussed in Chapter 4). Lobular cancer often produces very subtle changes in the breast that may be easily missed by the patient, the doctor, and the mammogram. In many cases, the first signs of cancer are due to distant metastases.

We approach the patient with Stage IV breast cancer differently from patients with Stage I, II, and III disease. In patients with earlier stage disease, the goal is to *cure* the patient by destroying all visible disease within the breast and the lymph nodes with the addition of adjuvant drug treatment.

In patients diagnosed with Stage IV disease, the possibility of cure is much lower, and the goal of treatment is to prolong the life of the patient by keeping her in remission for as long as possible.

For patients with Stage IV disease, the care team's responsibility is:

- to improve the patient's quality of life by relieving symptoms caused by the cancer;
- to prolong disease-free and symptom-free survival;
- to prevent and treat complications of the cancer;
- to minimize side effects of cancer treatment; and
- to relieve distress and support the patient and her family throughout her journey.

Unlike early-stage breast cancer, in which surgery is employed first, patients with Stage IV cancer are generally prescribed drug treatment as the first line of defense. Since the disease is systemic, they need systemic treatment.

Depending on the type of breast cancer, systemic treatment can be as simple as an estrogen-blocking agent ("hormone therapy"), one or more of the large number of active chemotherapy drugs, a targeted agent such as trastuzumab, or a combination of these drugs.

There are many very effective treatments available for patients with Stage IV disease.

Below are our first priorities when caring for a patient with Stage IV disease:

1. First, we assess the symptoms that the cancer is causing and take steps to relieve them; doctors call this process *palliation,* which means relief of symptoms. Sometimes this will require radiation (to relieve pain caused by bone metastases, for example), or even surgery (if a patient has a large amount of fluid collecting in the abdomen causing severe pain).

2. The second priority is to treat the disease with drug treatment appropriate to the type of cancer with the goal of killing the cancer and achieving *remission* (in which all visible tumor has been destroyed).

3. The third goal is to *maintain* the patient in remission for as long as possible.

4. And the final goal is to support the patient and family through the treatment process, which can be physically arduous, emotionally stressful, and expensive.

It is important to emphasize that most women with Stage IV breast cancer can achieve control of their disease, with appropriate medical treatment, and significantly prolong their lives, often for years.

Every Treatment Plan Is Unique

A final word or two on the subject of treatment choices: This book is intended to help inform women and their caregivers about breast cancer and its possible treatments. Only the doctors who have examined you and reviewed all of the relevant tests can give you *specific* treatment advice.

It is very important for patients to understand the forms of treatment available so that you feel comfortable talking with your team of doctors and can work with them to determine the best treatment plan based on facts, not on fears. After all, it is your body and your life, and you have every right to understand your treatment options. No one expects you to know as much as your doctors, but you have to know enough to feel comfortable with and stick with the treatment program they lay out for you.

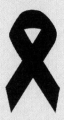

Metastatic Breast Cancer Is a Highly Treatable Condition

IN 2004, A VERY ACTIVE CHRISTINE STEWART, age fifty-six, noticed that her breast was sore and swollen. "I thought that it could be something else," she says, "and *hoped* it was something else. So I put it off for about four months. Then one morning I woke up, and my right arm was very sore underneath."

Christine found a plum-sized lump under her arm. Her last screening mammogram had been done *three years* earlier and was reportedly normal. When she went for an appointment and her doctor saw the large tumor in her breast, he recommended immediate surgery. Christine chose to come to CTCA for a second opinion.

When I first examined her in October 2004, I found her right breast to be massively enlarged, with a six-centimeter mass under her right arm. Multiple liver metastases were found on CAT scans; her breast biopsy found an ER-positive, HER2neu-negative invasive ductal carcinoma. Christine had a tough road ahead; she clearly had Stage IV disease.

Christine was treated initially with chemotherapy, which produced excellent shrinkage of all of her tumors. Despite this aggressive treatment, she never felt or looked sick. Eventually she underwent a right mastectomy with removal of her axillary nodes. (She decided against reconstruction, which she later regretted. "It's hard to have one breast during swimsuit season!" she told us.)

It was then that her treatment became a little unconventional. With such a large tumor mass and axillary nodes involved, she clearly required postmastectomy radiation to the chest wall and axilla. Because of the initial liver involvement, however, our radiation specialists developed an innovative treatment plan designed specifically for her.

After further chemotherapy, she was placed on a simple hormone-blocking pill, which she continues to take on a daily basis. The result? Christine achieved a complete remission of her cancer, which has persisted now for approximately eight years.

When I saw her last in August 2013, she remained apparently cancer-free and was enjoying life to the fullest.

"The best thing women can do for themselves is have regular mammograms," Christine says. "I was very irregular with mine, and I regret that. And you can't assume that doctors know all the answers. Ask questions, take control, and be empowered."

Doctor's Comments

Patients with advanced breast cancer should not view their situation as hopeless. Patients and their doctors have to remember that there are many very effective treatments available. It is also crucial to remember that there is no "one-size-fits-all" approach to treatment.

Christine's story illustrates a very important lesson, namely that when patients respond well to drug treatment for advanced disease, it opens up many additional treatment options.

A "one-size-fits-all approach" no longer exists. Every patient is unique and needs a personalized treatment plan, based on the specific details of her disease and tailored to her individual characteristics. Modern breast cancer treatment frequently uses all three major modalities: surgery, radiation, and drug treatment.

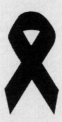

The Value of Neo-Adjuvant Therapy

IN MAY 2011, WHEN EVA ARROYO'S FOSTER DAUGHTER was sick in the hospital, Eva picked her up and held her close to her chest. Suddenly she felt a sharp pain in her left breast—one that almost took her breath away. A very faithful person, Eva immediately began praying and talking to God. She knew she had cancer.

Because she was caring for her daughter, Eva initially ignored the lump and pain in her breast. Two months later, she called her doctor for an order for a mammogram. As soon as the mammogram was completed, she asked for an ultrasound and a biopsy, all in the same day.

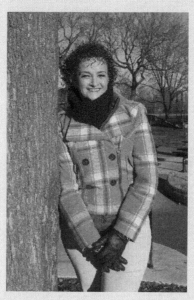

"It's only cancer. It's just a word. You can't let fear control you.
Now I laugh more, I don't worry so much, and I feel blessed every day."
— *Eva Arroyo*

"The next day, I called my doctor and asked her to tell me the results," Eva says. "I knew that I had cancer, but that everything would be OK."

Eva was diagnosed with a fast-growing Stage II cancer. Her doctors recommended a mastectomy. When she came to CTCA for a second opinion, she expressed the desire to avoid mastectomy, if at all possible.

When I first examined Eva, her left breast contained a large mass, approximately three centimeters in diameter. Because the tumor was HER2neu positive, we were confident that we could shrink it significantly with chemotherapy and trastuzumab.

Eva agreed, and after two treatments, the tumor mass in the breast could no longer be felt. Eva agreed to have breast-conserving surgery early in November 2011. At that time, a pathologic study revealed only microscopic residual cancer in her breast.

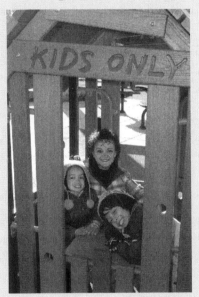

She received additional chemotherapy and radiation after surgery and completed one year of adjuvant trastuzumab in November 2012. During follow-up examinations, Eva remains cancer-free.

Because of her excellent response to preoperative chemotherapy, Eva was able to avoid mastectomy, and her prognosis for complete cure is excellent.

Throughout this journey, Eva relied on her faith to carry her through. "It's only cancer," she says. "It's just a word. You can't let fear control you. I refused to give it power. I put my faith in the power of God. Now I laugh more, I don't worry so much, and I feel blessed every day."

Doctor's Comments

Eva's story is very illuminating in that she did not accept the initial recommendation for immediate mastectomy and instead sought additional options.

Because of the biologic nature of her cancer (HER2neu positive), she was an ideal candidate for trastuzumab-based chemotherapy. With an excellent response to preoperative drug treatment, the tumor shrank significantly, thus allowing much more limited surgery.

Note that none of these options was offered to her initially. It is very important that every patient with breast cancer have a consultation with a qualified medical oncologist and a surgeon before any treatment is started.

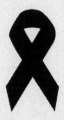

Cancer doesn't have to be horrible.

WHEN MARIE BOTCHIE WAS THIRTY-FIVE, her doctor suggested she have a baseline mammogram since her mother had a history of uterine cancer and her aunt had a history of breast cancer. When Marie received a regular mammogram at forty, her doctor noticed what he thought were calcium deposits.

"We really didn't see tumors," she says, "and the doctor thought there was only a 10 percent chance it was cancer. But if I hadn't had a baseline mammogram, the cancer wouldn't have been detected at all."

A subsequent biopsy of the breast led to the detection of invasive ductal carcinoma in her right breast. The Stage IIIB tumor sitting against her chest wall was six centimeters in diameter. Her cancer, which was ER- and PR-positive, had invaded six of eleven of her right axillary nodes (the lymph nodes under her armpit).

Her oncologist suggested starting chemotherapy followed by radiation, and gave her a 49 percent chance of surviving past five years.

"On April 5, 2004, I smoked my last cigarette and had a good cry," Marie explained. "The next morning, I set out on a mission to make cancer the *best* thing to ever happen to me, not the *worst*."

Marie had both breasts surgically removed and chose not to have breast reconstruction. Soon thereafter, she came to CTCA. Because of the size of the primary tumor, and the presence of six positive lymph nodes, she was determined to be at very high risk for recurrence and received chemotherapy with three different medications to eliminate any residual cancer cells from her body. She received radiation therapy, had her ovaries removed (to reduce the impact of estrogen in her body), and took an aromatase inhibitor for five years to completely stop all estrogen production in her body.

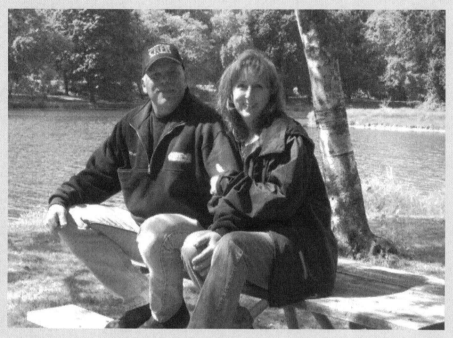

"There are not a lot of positive outcomes from resistance,
particularly when dealing with cancer."
— *Iva "Marie" Botchie, with her husband Michael*

Nearly ten years later, Marie has no evidence of cancer recurrence. Mild osteoporosis from the aromatase inhibitor is her only long-lasting side effect from treatment.

"Having cancer is almost like being turned wrong-side-out, given a few good shakes, and then put right-side-out again, all fresh and clean," Marie says. "Cancer doesn't have to be horrible. You can allow it to change your life in a positive way."

Doctor's Comments

Marie's experience is inspirational and also very educational. First, Stage III breast cancer is a highly treatable disease, but it requires a combination of surgery, radiation, and drug treatment. In Marie's case, we were able to take full advantage of the fact that her tumor was strongly estrogen dependent. Marie fully understood the rationale for the treatments we recommended and made the decision to move forward with great courage.

While never easy, it is important to emphasize that all patients newly diagnosed with breast cancer now have many options available to them.

One final point: Marie was diagnosed as having the BRCA mutation, although she did not fit the classic BRCA stereotype. She is not Jewish, her tumor was not triple negative, and she didn't have a strong family history. It was only after her mother developed ovarian cancer that she was tested for BRCA.

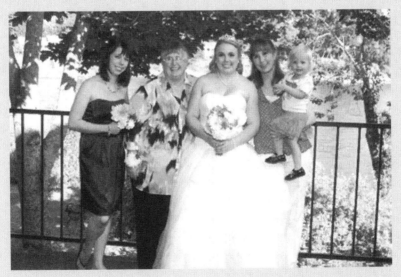

Marie holding her granddaughter at her daughter's wedding.

CHAPTER 8

With Knowledge Comes Power: Why Trust, Respect, and Communication Are Critical to Good Cancer Care

"I asked, 'Is there hope?' And the doctor looked me right in the eye and said, 'There is always hope.' In that moment, my whole life changed."
—Rosalind Landrum

Like any other relationship between two people, there are good ones and bad ones. So what makes a good doctor-patient relationship? And why is a good doctor-patient relationship so important?

We all bring to the table a lifetime of experiences that shape and influence our worldview and decision-making processes. Our past experiences with modern medicine have left impressions on us in terms of our confidence, our ability to handle stress, our level of trust in others, and our faith in the future.

All of these intangible factors play a significant role in how patients view their disease and treatment. They influence whether a patient will seek a diagnosis as soon as she feels a breast lump and whether she'll trust and accept her doctor's treatment recommendations.

As a doctor, my goal is to educate and guide the patient to make the most appropriate choices so that she may receive the best possible treatment for her particular condition. After all, the focus is *always* on the patient and her welfare. To do that, I must earn her trust and respect, and I must be able to clearly communicate and educate her about her condition and what we can do to successfully treat it.

Trust

The hope is that you can find a doctor in whom you can trust. You have to trust that he or she is knowledgeable about your medical condition and is giving you the best possible medical advice.

You can be pretty confident (and it is easy to check) that all of your doctors are Board certified in their particular specialty, which means that they have demonstrated a basic level of competence in treating patients with breast cancer. But there is much more to being a good doctor than being clinically competent. You must be confident that your doctor has *your* best interests at heart. This is especially true of medical systems in which doctors are paid for *activity*, and not paid (or paid much less) for withholding treatment.

There are times when decisions regarding treatment options are not always clear cut—when several options may be equally appropriate. The patient has every right to fully understand, not only *what* her doctor is recommending but also *why*, as well as what other choices are available.

Like any other relationship, you have to listen to your instincts. If you don't feel comfortable with your doctor, then he or she isn't the right doctor for you.

Statistical Proof: Trust Matters

I recently conducted a study of thirty patients who either delayed consulting a medical doctor, despite having obvious cancers, or refused all conventional treatment (surgery, radiation, and drug treatment) after biopsies confirmed that they did indeed have breast cancer. Instead of receiving appropriate medical treatment, they embarked on what turned out to be unsuccessful attempts at controlling their diseases, exclusively through a variety of alternative measures. These alternatives included a macrobiotic diet, fruit and vegetable juices, organic foods, yoga, meditation, radioactive stones, vitamins, chelation, and other unproven methods of treatment.

After their experiments with alternative treatments failed to control their diseases, they came to CTCA. By then, most of them had very advanced disease, and complete cure was no longer possible. In our study, we wanted to understand why these thirty patients had made the initial decision to forgo conventional treatment despite an obvious cancer diagnosis. Why did they choose some pretty bizarre "treatments" that had no obvious scientific basis?

Each patient was interviewed by a compassionate and experienced clinical psychologist, who also interviewed thirty control subjects. The control group was comprised of patients with breast cancer who did not reject conventional medical treatments, but were treated at our institution at the time of initial diagnosis with a program of surgery, radiation, and drug treatment. As is our standard practice, these patients also received recommendations from our complementary and integrative medicine team.

What came out of these interviews was a startling conclusion. **Almost all of the thirty patients in our study who refused conventional treatment felt rejected and disrespected by their original physicians, after they expressed an interest or belief in and asked questions about integrative medicine.**

As a result of their doctors' negative reactions, they rejected ALL conventional cancer treatment (surgery, radiation, and chemotherapy), and instead they embraced a variety of alternative treatments that *by themselves* were incapable of preventing the progression of their disease.

In most cases, that decision resulted in potentially curable cancers progressing to an advanced stage—and no longer curable.

When questioned by our psychologist, the patients stated that when they expressed an interest in integrative therapies, their doctors became angry or hostile and expressed very negative statements, such as, "If you do this, you'll never see your children grow up."

And so these patients, who were already oriented toward holistic health care, reacted to their physicians' attitudes by refusing potentially curative treatment and instead sought alternative therapy only, with disastrous results.

The important message for doctors and other health care professionals from this study is this: Whether or not you agree with your patient's point of view, you have to be supportive and show appropriate respect for her opinions.

Communication

Trust, respect, and communication are intertwined. Without mutual trust and respect, there cannot be good communication. And without good communication, there cannot be good patient care.

It is important that patients trust their doctors, but trust is not the same as blind faith. You have every right to fully understand, not only what your doctor is recommending for you but also *why* he or she is making those recommendations. A good doctor understands this and respects your right to ask questions and their obligation to answer those questions fully. No reasonable doctor expects you to accept his or her recommendations without a full explanation of the rationale for those recommendations.

Today, it is a given that the patient be provided all of the information relevant to her medical situation. But this was not always the case. When I was a medical student in the United Kingdom forty years ago, we never told patients that they had cancer. We used vague terms like "inflammation" or "abnormality." Sure, every woman knew that she wasn't losing her breast because of some minor issue (in those days mastectomy was the rule). But the word *cancer* was never uttered. We assumed that patients couldn't handle the truth. That paternalistic approach is now rightly considered archaic, yet some health care practitioners still have trouble communicating clearly with their patients.

Poor doctor-patient communication can cause serious problems. Several years ago, a young woman named Jean came to CTCA. Jean was thirty-seven, and she had breast cancer that had spread throughout her bones and liver. When I reviewed Jean's records, I saw that she had not received any chemotherapy after her breast surgery. When I asked her about this, she said that her surgeon had recommended chemotherapy, but when Jean told the surgeon that she was afraid of the side effects, the surgeon simply shrugged and left the room. No one made the effort to explain to Jean *why* chemotherapy was needed, and there was no further discussion of the subject. Jean recovered from her surgery, but two years later the cancer returned.

The good news is that Jean has responded very well to chemotherapy, is now in stable remission, and is enjoying life with her husband and young children.

Jean's story is an example of very poor doctor-patient communication—an extreme example, perhaps, but by no means unique.

Don't Be Afraid to Ask Questions

In July 2010, the *Wall Street Journal* described a study from the Centers for Disease Control and Prevention that reported that *nearly nine out of ten adults* had difficulty following medical advice because it was largely incomprehensible to them.

Too often doctors use medical jargon that patients just don't understand. Numerous studies have shown that patients who do not fully comprehend what their doctors tell them are much more likely to skip necessary medical tests, fail to take medications properly, and have much poorer outcomes as a result.

I can't tell you how many times I've listened to younger doctors "explain" the medical facts to patients who are clearly mystified by what they are hearing, but are just too intimidated to ask questions. Please, if you don't understand what you've just heard from your doctor, ask the doctor to explain it in simpler terms.

Communication Must Be Two Way

Please remember that doctors are not mind readers; you have to tell your doctor everything that's going on. As crazy as it sounds, many patients don't like to complain if they don't feel well. They think the doctor will get angry or upset with them. They will tell the nurse how they really feel, but oftentimes, they are very reluctant to tell the doctor. But it is in your best interest to provide your doctor with all of the facts about your medical condition.

Seeking treatment for cancer can be intimidating for anyone. After all, having cancer is a terrifying experience, and you're dependent on the doctor to work with you to restore your health.

Do not hesitate to ask your doctor questions or express doubts or reservations about his or her treatment recommendation. Good doctors understand that patients and their families may be intimidated or frightened and will do their best to make them feel at ease.

The best doctors and health care systems understand how important it is to *empower* their patients—to emphasize that the patient has the right to fully understand her disease and the treatment that is being recommended and that she will not be judged for having an opinion.

As a physician, it is not my job to "tell" my patients what to do. Rather, it is to give them all the relevant facts and guide them to make what I believe are the best decisions for their individual situations. Modern breast cancer treatment is complicated, and that's why you should make notes of what you want to ask your doctor before you get together and also take notes of what information you're given. Believe me, no reasonable doctor will object to you taking notes or recording your conversation.

We all know that in today's health care climate, there are economic and other pressures on doctors to rush patients through the system. But it is critical that there is adequate *time* devoted for effective communication between doctor and patient. I'm fortunate to work in an institution that recognizes the importance of providing adequate time for the patient to meet with all members of the health care team. If you feel rushed during your doctor appointments, or feel that the doctor is impatient with you, then you're not getting the care that you need and deserve.

Modern treatment of breast cancer requires the efforts of a whole team, so doctor-to-doctor communication is vitally important throughout the process of diagnosis and treatment. At Cancer Treatment Centers of America, all of the principles we have outlined in this chapter form the basis of what we call the **Patient Empowered Care® Model.**

The foundation of patient empowerment is the idea that the patient and her welfare are the primary focus of all of our efforts. Every patient has the right to have all of her concerns addressed and to fully understand all of the details of her medical condition and treatment plan that her health care team has recommended. Our team will take as much time as necessary to explain, not only *what* treatment is recommended and the alternatives that are available but also *why* specific recommendations have been made.

The empowered patient understands that the choice of treatment is hers, and whatever choices she makes and opinions she expresses will be treated with respect. Indeed, throughout her CTCA experience, we ensure that every patient will be treated respectfully.

Patient Empowered Care®

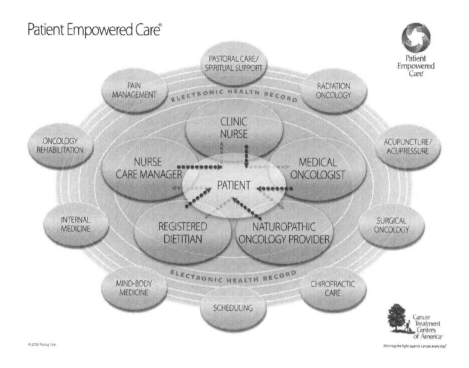

It is unreasonable to expect any patient, especially the newly diagnosed patient with cancer who is invariably frightened, to make rational decisions about treatment if she is not fully informed of all the relevant medical facts. An empathetic health care professional who takes the time to address all patient concerns can really be life saving. One hour spent explaining to a patient and her family the details of her breast cancer and the treatment options available to her (with DIAGRAMS!) is absolutely essential for the patient who needs to make the correct treatment choices.

Too many doctors don't recognize the value of this time, and too often the task of educating the patient is delegated to a more junior member of the health care team.

But there is much more to CTCA care than simply educating the patient. The entire focus at CTCA is on the patient and her welfare.

Patient Empowered Care Model

It is the responsibility of the entire health care team to:

- educate the patient as to the facts of her situation;

- address all of her concerns;

- explain her diagnosis and prognosis in plain terms that she can understand (no false hope but no unwarranted threats or pessimism);

- encourage her to ask questions and take the time to answer those questions;

- provide a professional, caring environment in which the patient feels comfortable expressing her feelings;

- take the time to establish a mutually respectful and trusting relationship with the patient and her family;

- guide the patient to make the correct treatment choices; and

- ensure a positive relationship with the patient throughout treatment and beyond.

We believe that it is important to provide an environment of hope, optimism, and caring for every patient.

The Importance of Emotional Support: Realism and Hope

When I begin to treat any patient with advanced breast cancer, I don't know how well she will respond to treatment. I may know that approximately 60 percent of patients I have previously treated with a specific program of drugs responded well with significant tumor shrinkage. But my previous experience and the medical literature don't allow me to state with any certainty whether *any individual patient* will respond to treatment, nor how completely she will respond or for how long.

In that respect, the medical treatment of a patient with advanced breast cancer is fundamentally different from the treatment of patients with noncancerous conditions. The doctor treating a patient with diabetes or high blood pressure can be pretty confident that his or her patient will respond to medical treatment.

In contrast, the current state of the science of oncology is such that we don't have accurate predictors of response for most chemotherapy drugs. The only way to determine how beneficial a treatment will be for any individual patient is to actually *give* that treatment and observe the effect.

Given the uncertainties involved in modern breast cancer treatment, it is totally inappropriate to warn the patient of a poor prognosis, and certainly inappropriate to make predictions of how long they are going to live even before they have started treatment. And yet, patient after patient tells me the dire "deadlines" that other doctors have predicted for them.

When any woman is starting what is likely to be a long and sometimes difficult journey, she needs encouragement and support, not pessimism. I sincerely believe that the positive, optimistic, caring attitude that every CTCA patient experiences is much more likely to be beneficial than a negative or pessimistic one.

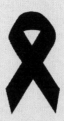

Trust and Respect Are Essential for Good Patient Care

IN 2003, CAROL STRAMOWSKI JUST DIDN'T FEEL WELL. She knew something was wrong. During her last pregnancy, twenty years earlier, she'd had an inflamed breast, so she'd always kept an eye on it.

Carol went for a mammogram in October, but nothing showed up. In January, still feeling poorly, Carol had another mammogram that detected a three-centimeter mass. A biopsy confirmed that she had infiltrating lobular carcinoma. The tumor was ER/PR strongly positive and HER2neu negative.

In February, Carol had a left mastectomy. While waiting to begin chemotherapy treatments, the cancer recurred, and in March, she had a right mastectomy.

Thankfully, Carol says, she had a wonderful oncologist who gave her some very good advice. "Be your own advocate," the oncologist said. "Get copies of your files and do some research. Don't be led." These words stuck with Carol.

In April, Carol was started on adjuvant chemotherapy that included four cycles of doxorubicin and one cycle of docetaxel. Her oncologist suggested she take tamoxifen, but she declined. "I was convinced the drugs were killing me," she says.

Two years later, in July 2006, the cancer recurred in her left mastectomy scar. The cancer was excised, and Carol received radiation therapy. In March 2007, Carol was offered an aromotase inhibitor (anastrazole), but again, she declined.

Four years later in 2011, another recurrence in her left mastectomy scar was excised. And that's when Carol came to CTCA and became my patient.

At CTCA, we started Carol on anastrazole, a hormone-blocking treatment, to keep her cancer at bay. Carol continues this therapy and is able to tolerate it well. Our breast cancer team continues to support her to make sure that side effects are kept to a minimum and to address all of her concerns on an ongoing basis.

"My advice to other women is: get a second or even a third opinion," Carol says. "Do your homework, and learn to be an advocate for yourself. Don't rush into three or four kinds of treatment, but also don't be stubborn. Follow your doctor's advice to the letter!"

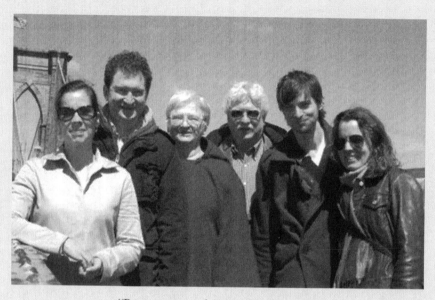

"Be your own advocate. Don't be led."
— *Carol Stramowski, center, with her family*

Doctor's Comments

Lobular carcinoma is frequently highly estrogen sensitive, and hormone-blocking therapy is very effective in preventing recurrence and controlling recurrent disease.

When I asked Carol why she initially declined hormone treatment, she told me that in 2004, her oncologist had told her, "If you don't take the tamoxifen, then you're an idiot!" And that unfortunate experience was still resonating with her in 2007 when she had a recurrence of her disease and once again refused hormone-blocking treatment.

That is why mutual respect and good patient-doctor communication are so critical. When I first met Carol in 2011, we spent a significant amount of time discussing the rationale for hormone treatment and why I strongly recommended it. Once Carol fully understood the reasons and benefits, she readily agreed.

As a doctor, I can't think of a better use of my time. The potential benefits of hormone treatment for a patient with even widespread lobular cancer of the breast are significant.

CHAPTER 9

Common Patient and Doctor Errors in Breast Cancer Treatment and How to Avoid Them

*"Cancer care can seem like you're in a maze.
You have to choose whom you trust very carefully.
And you might have to leave town to find the best treatment."*
—*Kim Niernberger*

A good doctor-patient relationship is *essential* because breast cancer is always a potentially fatal disease. And treatment is often required for years.

In my experience, the more patients understand the rationale for cancer treatment and the details of that treatment, the more likely they are to make good treatment choices and complete the treatment plan.

And when doctors do a poor job explaining treatment options to a patient, or appear impatient or hostile toward patients when they ask questions or express an interest in alternative medicine, that's when patients are more likely to make the wrong decisions (see following table).

It isn't just a matter of providing patients with the medical facts, however. It is important that every doctor builds a relationship of trust with his or her patient.

Common Patient Errors in the Treatment of Breast Cancer

1. Patients refuse all conventional treatment, opting instead for alternative treatments alone.

2. Patients refuse part of a recommended course of treatment (usually chemotherapy and/or hormones) after surgery.

3. Patients demand excessive or overtreatment (usually complete or bilateral mastectomy where more limited surgery would be just as effective).

4. Patients end a course of treatment prematurely.

The previous chapter included results from a study of thirty patients who refused all conventional treatment for recently diagnosed breast cancer. In that study, we found that almost every one of these women had a similar experience: when they expressed an interest in integrative medicine, their doctors became hostile, angry, and impatient with them.

When the women in the study came to CTCA, generally with advanced disease, all but one of the thirty readily accepted conventional cancer treatment.

It's hard to avoid the conclusion that a more sympathetic and open-minded approach with these patients at the time of first diagnosis might have produced a more favorable outcome.

Doctor Errors That Lead to Patients Choosing Inappropriate Treatment

- Not listening to the patient
- Showing a lack of respect or being dismissive of the patient's beliefs or wishes
- Allocating inadequate time and/or showing lack of patience and kindness
- Refusing to discuss integrative treatment options
- Poor communication skills
- Threatening the patient with dire consequences if she doesn't follow the doctor's advice
- Rushing the patient to make immediate treatment decisions

You'll notice that the issues listed above are not due to doctors *recommending* or *using* the wrong treatment. Most cancer specialists are well trained and competent in making treatment decisions. It's usually a problem of *attitude* and *communication*.

Good communication is critical from the time of first diagnosis and must continue throughout a patient's course of treatment. Consider this hypothetical situation:

Imagine a patient who had a tumor removed from her breast in January, and then had five months of adjuvant chemotherapy. She's just finished nearly two months of radiation to her breast, and her hair is starting to come back. She's been through a pretty tough eight months. She sees her oncologist, who tells her it is time to start five years of a hormone pill that will give her hot flashes and weight gain. Five years?!

"Why do I need that?" the patient invariably asks. "The surgeon told me she got it all, and I've gone through all this chemo and radiation!"

Don't you agree that this patient deserves a respectful, detailed discussion with her doctor *in terms that she can understand* of the reasons for additional therapy? Of course she does! And she also needs repeated encouragement to continue taking the medicine throughout the next five years (or longer).

It is hardly surprising that many studies have shown a very significant rate of patient noncompliance, meaning that women opt out of some or all of their treatment programs. In some studies, for example, *more than half* of the women who were recommended five years of estrogen-blocking treatment stopped prematurely.

Over the past several years, we have studied how often patients with early-stage breast cancer followed the treatment programs recommended by their cancer doctors:

- We looked at all patients with recurrent breast cancer over a three-year period (from July 2009 through June 2012) who were initially treated for early-stage breast cancer at other hospitals.
- Despite the treatment they received, their cancer recurred, and they came to CTCA for treatment.
- In contrast to the previous study of thirty patients who refused all conventional cancer treatment, these patients had received conventional cancer treatment (a combination of surgery, radiation, drug treatment, chemotherapy, and/or hormones).
- We reviewed all of their initial treatment to evaluate whether their original treatment was adequate and met current national guidelines for the treatment of early breast cancer.
- These guidelines were developed by a panel of experts, the National Comprehensive Cancer Network (NCCN). The guidelines are constantly updated and are widely available on the Internet.

Noncompliance Leads to Poor Results

The results of our study were very revealing. Over a three-year period we saw 382 patients whose breast cancer recurred despite previous treatment for what was early, potentially curable disease. Of those 382 patients, 188 (47 percent) did not complete the recommended treatment. That's nearly half of the patients treated!

That study confirms what other breast cancer doctors have found, namely that many women treated for early breast cancer frequently don't follow the treatment recommendations that they receive. It also suggests that this noncompliance may well be an important reason why these patients were not cured.

Why do patients refuse cancer treatment? Fear and lack of knowledge are to blame.

Ironically, it's the patient with early stage breast cancer who is more likely to refuse treatment. These are the very patients in whom refusal of treatment can cause the greatest harm by reducing the patient's chances of complete cure of her disease.

Why do so many patients with early stage breast cancer refuse conventional treatment? I believe the answer is a combination of fear and lack of knowledge.

Fear is absolutely understandable in any patient with cancer. Being told you have cancer must be one of the most frightening experiences a person can have. It is natural to be afraid of the unknown, afraid of dying, and afraid of the pain and physical suffering that are often associated with advanced cancer. **But early stage breast cancer is a curable disease!**

Patients are most afraid of drug treatment (chemotherapy and hormone-blockers). Although patients are naturally apprehensive about surgery, they are generally much more likely to accept the need for surgery than other types of cancer treatment.

In the study of 382 patients referred to earlier, nearly every patient completed the surgical treatment that was recommended. This is hardly surprising since surgery has been recognized as the primary treatment for cancer for centuries. Breast surgery also is seen by the patient as a clearly defined event, with limited potential for major side effects. Once you've had the surgery, it's over. There's a certain simple logic to cutting out the diseased area that patients can easily understand.

Radiation is also usually accepted by most patients because it is directed to the area where the disease was first identified (the breast and node-bearing areas). Most patients understand the logic of using radiation as an additional form of local treatment after surgery. Radiation is also given for a few weeks only. So, like surgery, radiation is generally accepted by the patient as a short-term measure directed against the local site of disease.

When weighing the benefits of treatment versus the risks, the decision to recommend radiation treatment is generally an easy one to make. Less than one in a thousand patients develop a severe complication from radiation, and most women benefit by reducing the risk of recurrence of their cancer and significantly increasing the cure rate.

In general, when patients with breast cancer refuse some form of treatment, it is usually drug treatment (chemotherapy and hormone therapy). There are several reasons for this.

First, many patients have an exaggerated idea of the toxicity and side effects associated with drug treatment for cancer, especially chemotherapy, but also estrogen-blocking, "hormone" treatment.

Second, in contrast with surgery and radiation, drug treatment requires a significant time commitment from the patient, extending over months or years. Chemotherapy is usually given for four or five months after surgery, while hormone-blocking treatment is generally recommended for five years or longer.

Because it is almost always drug treatment that the patient with early breast cancer refuses, it is really the responsibility of the medical oncologist to fully explain the rationale for and the details of their proposed treatment and to encourage patients to stick with the proposed treatment plan.

Risks and Benefits of Drug Treatment

When considering any cancer treatment, doctors have to evaluate and strike a balance between the *risks* and *benefits* of treatment.

Most people don't understand just how effective and well tolerated modern cancer treatment can be. **We are so much better at treating patients with cancer today than we were in the past. And that means more *effective* treatment, and also *much less toxicity* (side effects) from treatment.**

Think how cell phones and computers have changed in the past twenty years. It is exactly the same with cancer treatment; there have been major technological advances. What you may have seen or heard of a relative's experience even ten years ago has little relevance to what you can expect today.

Dispelling the Myths of Today's Cancer Treatment

We have already discussed the advances that have been made to alleviate the nausea and vomiting after receiving chemotherapy. Today, vomiting due to chemotherapy is a thing of the past.

It is very important that doctors fully explain to their patients the rationale for adjuvant therapy, namely that the treatment she has been recommended is designed to reduce her risk of future cancer recurrence. Adjuvant treatment (both chemotherapy and hormone treatment) is usually used after all obvious disease has been surgically removed from the breast. Such treatment is directed against any microscopic disease that may remain after surgery.

The concept of taking potentially toxic medication to reduce the risk of a future negative event (disease recurrence) is a difficult one for some patients to accept. It requires a lot of explanation and constant encouragement. While the patient is receiving treatment (and experiencing side effects), it is not as if she can actually see or feel that the treatment is doing its job. In fact, the opposite may be true: the patient who refuses adjuvant treatment usually feels better than the patient receiving such treatment. After all, no treatment, no side effects, right?

Surgical Overtreatment

I do want to mention one other important issue—surgical overtreatment. Quite often, women come to us demanding bilateral mastectomies for what is early stage disease in one breast only. I've even seen patients with a small area of DCIS only (preinvasive cancer) demand a bilateral mastectomy. "I don't want to have to worry about my breasts ever again," is the refrain.

While that may be an entirely understandable emotional reaction, it is not in most patients' best interests to undergo such radical and unnecessary surgery. **The scientific data is clear; women who choose limited (breast-conserving) surgery are just as likely to be cured as those women who choose mastectomy.**

There are many women who demand and many surgeons who still recommend, not only removal of the affected breast but also the opposite breast, even though it is perfectly healthy and in all probability will stay healthy and noncancerous throughout the patient's life! If anything, this phenomenon has become more common in recent years.

To avoid excessive surgery, it is very important that women newly diagnosed with breast cancer fully understand what their lifetime risk is for developing a second cancer in the opposite breast. Many studies have shown that women newly diagnosed with breast cancer often have an exaggerated view of the probability of developing a second cancer in the opposite breast.

I would strongly recommend that before any woman agrees to or requests a prophylactic removal of the second breast, she gets an accurate prediction of her lifetime risk for a second cancer. In my opinion, the only situations in which prophylactic mastectomy should be considered is in the patient with documented BRCA gene mutation or other rare gene mutation in which breast cancer risk is high, and women who received previous radiation for Hodgkin Disease. These special situations are discussed later in Chapter 14.

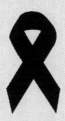

Biopsies Are Critical for Accurate Diagnosis

CARRIE FREEMAN WAS ONLY THIRTY-SEVEN in 2006 when she felt a spot on her right breast that just didn't feel right. A screening mammogram showed an abnormality, and an ultrasound revealed a nine-millimeter solid mass. The surgeon reassured Carrie that it was nothing and no biopsy was required, despite her mother's history of ovarian cancer and leukemia. He suggested a follow-up visit in six months.

During the next six months, Carrie became pregnant with her fourth child, and the mass in her right breast continued to grow. Her breast became inflamed, and she was given antibiotics four times.

In July 2007, one full year later, Carrie finally had a biopsy that confirmed ER/PR-positive breast cancer. She underwent neo-adjuvant chemotherapy to reduce the size of the nine-centimeter mass before surgery, and then had a bilateral mastectomy with radiation. All eight of the nodes under her right arm were positive for cancer, and the cancer had begun to spread in other directions.

She then had radiation to the right mastectomy site, axilla, and supraclavicular areas.

Because her cancer was hormone sensitive, Carrie also had her uterus and ovaries removed in April 2008 and began taking oral letrozole.

Carrie first came to CTCA for treatment in August 2008. There was no obvious recurrent disease at that time and letrozole was continued. But in March 2009, we noted several new skin tumors on Carrie's chest wall. A chemotherapy pill was added to the letrozole, and the skin nodules quickly resolved.

Carrie had several other small tumor recurrences, including a tiny cancer deposit found in her appendix in May 2010.

Carrie's positive attitude helped her ride the tide of her cancer. When she was first diagnosed, her husband had just been laid off, she was pregnant, and they had three small children at home. Carrie was the primary breadwinner but had to quit working when she began treatment. Carrie and her husband eventually wrote a book called *Cancer and Finances* to help others facing financial challenges during cancer treatment. She and her husband gave it away to help others through the complexities of insurance, estate planning, financial resources for copays, travel, hotels, and other necessities. Carrie also wrote a children's book to help children when a parent is diagnosed and treated for cancer.

Despite a valiant battle, Carrie finally succumbed to her disease in July 2013.

Doctor's Comments

Carrie's story describes a major error by her surgeon in 2006. Despite the ultrasound showing a solid mass, no biopsy was recommended. This decision was made, despite an abnormal mammogram and a significant family history of cancer. Solid breast lesions MUST be biopsied, regardless of the age of the patient.

The correct diagnosis was only made one year later, after a delay during which her ER-positive tumor was stimulated by pregnancy hormones. At that time Carrie was diagnosed with locally advanced (Stage III) disease.

As a result, her disease recurred in 2009, despite appropriate treatment in 2007 and 2008.

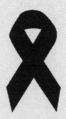

Follow Your Doctor's Treatment Recommendation

KIMBERLY NIERNBERGER FOUND A LUMP in her right breast when she was just thirty-five. A biopsy confirmed the diagnosis of invasive breast cancer.

Kim traveled to Kansas City, four hours away, for treatment of her Stage II breast cancer. In March 2003, she had a right lumpectomy in which the cancer and a margin of healthy tissue were removed, as were the lymph nodes beneath her right arm, to check them for cancer. Most were negative, but the cancer had spread to a few. In a second surgery in May 2003, a mastectomy was performed, and Kim received an implant.

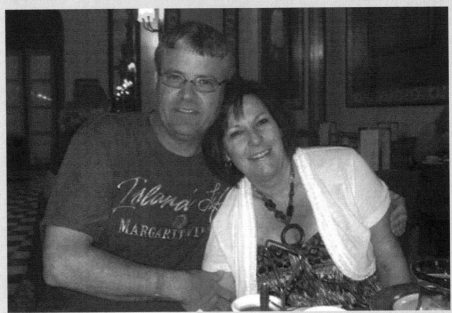

"I learned that I'm a lot stronger than I thought I was.
And I learned that I could do what doctors told me to do but still be empowered."
— Kim Niernberger, with her husband Darren

Kim declined the chemotherapy that was recommended after surgery and instead consulted an herbalist who prescribed a course of herbal supplements. One year later, the cancer came back in her reconstructed right breast. The cancer was surgically removed, and the doctor recommended chemotherapy, which she refused once again.

"Here's what I thought happened to people with cancer: have chemo, feel sick, get really skinny, and then die," Kim says. She had read a lot about eating healthy to keep cancer at bay and under control and thought she could control it herself. As a very spiritual person, she put her health in God's hands.

Kim remained cancer free until June 2008, when she noticed masses in her right breast and along her chest wall. She waited until November 2008, when she began to feel short of breath again, to consult a physician. A CAT scan disclosed a large mass in her right breast, plus multiple nodules in her lungs and enlarged lymph nodes above her collarbone. The cancer had spread to her lungs. "The doctor said to me, 'If I got results like this, I'd take that trip I'd always dreamed of.' I was floored," Kim says.

And that's when she came to CTCA for the first time and became my patient. Clinical evaluation at that time confirmed a massive, ulcerated tumor in her right breast, along with multiple nodules around the larger tumor.

Kim began receiving chemotherapy and trastuzumab to shrink the tumors in her lungs and improve her breathing; her oxygen levels were dangerously low. She underwent chemotherapy every three weeks. "I was so surprised that I didn't get sick or throw up," she says. "I felt great, and I looked good, too!" Kim flew from Kansas to Chicago and home again each day she received treatment. Her only side effect was fatigue the day after each treatment.

This therapy completely resolved all disease in her breast and improved the lung nodules. She stayed in remission on trastuzumab alone for about eighteen months. Then, we found two new nodules in her right axilla (armpit); a CAT scan also showed progression of the lung nodules. Kim stopped taking trastuzumab and began taking two oral medications, lapatinib and capecitabine, which caused the tumor nodules in her axilla and most of the lung lesions to resolve. She's had some limited side effects from these powerful medications, but they are tolerable. And as of September 2013, she remains in excellent remission.

Kim's advice for other women: "Cancer care can seem like you're in a maze. Many women don't know that there are other options out there, and some are afraid to travel because of their kids, spouse, or the cost. But you have to choose in whom you trust very carefully. And you might have to leave town to find the best treatment. I learned that I'm a lot stronger than I thought I was. And I learned that I could do what doctors told me to do but still be empowered."

"It has been almost ten years since this journey began," Kim concludes. "I remember thinking, 'Who is going to raise my kids? Will I ever see them graduate or get married?' And now I've seen all that and more and look forward to meeting my first grandchild in April. Thanks to Dr. Citrin, CTCA, and God—life is so precious."

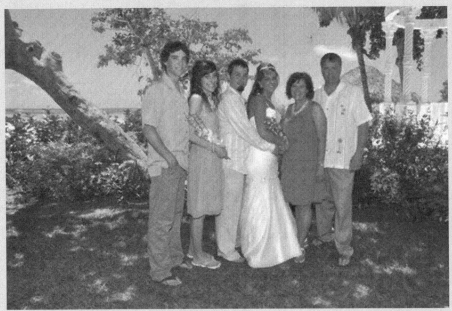

Doctor's Comments

Kim's experience demonstrates very clearly that partial treatment of breast cancer is not successful. Effective treatment of cancer requires the complete surgical removal of all evident disease, often combined with radiation and drug treatment indicated by the particular biology of the tumor.

In common with many of the patients referred to us, Kim had previously declined any drug treatment despite the aggressive nature of her tumor (HER2neu positive) and the development of disease recurrence in 2004.

It was only in 2008, when she had evident disease in the breast and extensive lung tumors were causing shortness of breath that she finally agreed to receive chemotherapy.

Almost five years later, Kim remains in an excellent remission. Kim's experience shows how a series of different drug treatments, based on the particular biologic characteristics of her disease, can be very effective.

CHAPTER 10

Can Breast Cancer Be Cured with Alternative Therapies?

"The treatments I endured before coming to CTCA were much worse and not effective. Surgery is no fun, believe me, but it was necessary because cancer isn't going to go away on its own!"
—Sandra Dillahunty

In addition to the established forms of treatment that doctors use—namely surgery, radiation, and drug treatment—many patients are also very interested to learn what natural or holistic measures *they themselves* can use to increase their chances of cure.

There are several reasons why patients with breast cancer are attracted to alternative treatments.

In its earliest stages, breast cancer does not produce disabling symptoms.

Some diseases produce very obvious symptoms that something is seriously wrong. For example, a person having a heart attack will usually have severe chest pains or shortness of breath. If you have a broken leg or are vomiting blood, there is no question that you are in trouble.

However, the patient with early stage breast cancer doesn't look or feel ill. Since her only complaint is usually the presence of a small, painless lump, she may not feel the same sense of urgency to seek medical care as someone suffering from a heart attack.

Breast cancer is a chronic illness, not an acute illness, so the patient has time to experiment with alternative treatments.

The term *acute* relates to how rapidly a disease evolves. *Acute* doesn't mean severe; it means a disease that is developing rapidly. Heart attack and pneumonia are referred to as *acute* illnesses. Patients get sick suddenly, and effective treatment is needed right away. The same is true of a patient who needs urgent surgery for appendicitis or an attack of gallstones.

With *acute illnesses,* the timeline from start to finish is short, often measured in hours or days. With *chronic* illnesses, the disease continues over weeks, months, or even years. Examples of chronic diseases include diabetes, arthritis, high blood pressure, and breast cancer.

Although breast cancer is a very serious disease that can be life threatening, it usually takes months or even years for significant progression of the disease to become evident. To put it bluntly, most breast cancers don't kill the patient in days or even weeks (and certainly not in hours!). The chronic nature of the disease offers an opportunity for those who wish to explore natural treatments as an alternative to conventional therapies.

Conventional cancer treatments frequently produce unwanted side effects.

Chemotherapy, in particular, had a very bad reputation in the past for causing severe toxicity. The idea of using a gentler, natural treatment as an alternative to chemotherapy is very attractive.

Every health care professional who treats women with breast cancer acknowledges that, even with all the advances that have been made in the past forty years, some treatments can still cause significant side effects. If there were an easy, safe, natural, nontoxic treatment that could get rid of the cancer without the need for surgery, radiation, and drug treatment, it would indeed be wonderful!

A cancer diagnosis is frightening.

In addition to the very natural fear, many patients feel a sense of helplessness and dependency on strangers (their doctors). Patients ask me almost every day, "What can I do to help myself?" The idea of fighting cancer by changing your diet or taking a vitamin or herb is a very compelling one, especially if there is an "expert" telling you to avoid conventional cancer treatment and follow a natural approach.

Measures, such as regular exercise, not smoking, good nutrition, and meditation to promote emotional health, have been actively encouraged for many years.

Health and wellness movements have improved the health of the general population. It is only logical to expect the application of similar principles would benefit patients with cancer.

Many other medical conditions can be helped through holistic measures. Why not cancer?

Holistic health measures are often very helpful for patients with fibromyalgia, chronic fatigue, hypertension, and headache. And it would be wonderful if holistic treatments could be used to cure cancer. But, there is a world of difference between attempting to cure breast cancer with alternative treatments *alone* and *combining* the best of conventional cancer treatment with complementary medicine in an integrative, whole-body approach.

What is clear to experts who have extensively studied breast cancer is that effective treatment of breast cancer requires surgical removal of the abnormal (cancerous) tissue, often combined with radiation and drug treatment.

Consider these two patient stories.

Anna, a sixty-year-old African-American woman, was treated by a medical doctor who uses only herbs in his practice. She was seen in his office every month for three years until the tumor in her breast grew large enough to burst through the skin and caused severe pain and bleeding.

She then came to CTCA to be treated. I asked her, "What did your doctor say to you when he saw the tumor was obviously getting bigger?"

"He never examined me," she said. "I saw him for three years, and I never took my shirt off."

When her tumor began growing through the skin of her breast, Chris, a thirty-six-year-old woman from Cleveland, was led to believe the tumor's dramatic growth was a positive sign that the herbs and reflexology she was using were working. "That's excellent," she was told. "The cancer is leaving your body."

What's frightening is that I have met dozens of women with similar stories. I am not critical of Anna or Chris for using alternative treatments. I am critical of the "experts" who were trying to treat a disease they have no experience or training in treating, using wholly unproven methods of research that have no scientific basis. With nearly forty years of experience helping women fight breast cancer, I am also critical of any approach to treatment that does not rely on evidence-based, clinically proven methods of cancer treatment.

Breast cancer cannot be treated with holistic therapies alone.

A quick Internet search of the phrase "Alternative Therapy Breast Cancer" or "Natural Breast Cancer Treatment" will deliver millions of hits. *Millions.* Does that mean that the person who is newly diagnosed with breast cancer has millions of options available to her for treatment? In a word, no.

The Internet offers many websites that provide scientifically valid information from very reputable organizations and medical providers. Unfortunately, there are also many websites that assure readers they have the secret "cure" for cancer. They tell women with breast cancer that they don't need surgery, radiation, or any of the drug treatments, if they will only buy their natural "cancer cure."

How does a woman newly diagnosed with cancer sort out all of the information that is available? How can you tell what's genuine and what's not? In the following table is a list of the more popular alternative "treatments" that are promoted for patients with breast cancer.

Alternative "Treatments" for Breast Cancer

Alkaline water
Antineoplastons
Dietary manipulation (vegetarian, juicing, macrobiotics)
Essiac
Gerson method
Hydrazine
Hyperoxygenation therapies (hydrogen peroxide, ozone)
Antioxidants
Insulin-potentiated chemotherapy
Iscador (mistletoe)
Kelly/Gonzalez metabolic therapy
Laetrile (vitamin B17)
Livingston-Wheeler regimen
Metabolic therapy (including coffee enemas)
Simonton visualization techniques
Shark cartilage
High-dose, intravenous vitamin C

Websites that describe these and other natural cancer cures almost always contain one or more of the following elements:

1. The authors claim that they have discovered the single cause of cancer in the form of a fungus, worm, or bacterium that they or someone else identified many years ago. In all cases, it is something that is very clearly defined, like too much sugar.
2. Conventional medicine does not believe or accept their discovery.
3. There is often reference to chemical or biochemical terms, so it sounds scientifically impressive.
4. Conventional cancer treatment is often referred to in lurid terms ("Don't let them cut, slash, burn, poison you!").
5. The promoter of the natural cure has often been persecuted and prosecuted for offering his treatments because he/she is too successful. (Hence, their frequent locations in Mexico or small Caribbean Islands.) Most are not medical doctors.
6. The treatment offered by the website is not only simple, natural, and effective against almost all cancers but will also cure AIDS, fibromyalgia, arthritis, and many other diseases.
7. There are glowing testimonials from patients who were apparently cured of cancer by the product after conventional treatments left them feeling sick and weak (but no documentation of the details of their disease and recovery).
8. There is almost always a disclaimer at the end stating that what is offered should not in fact be considered as a recommended treatment for any medical condition.

Many of the websites and books that promote natural treatments for cancer sound authentic. So how do you sort out fact from fiction?

Ask the following questions:

1. What is the science behind the treatment that is being recommended? In other words, what is the scientific rationale for the treatment?
2. What is the clinical data that shows how effective the treatment has been in patients?
3. What training and experience in cancer medicine does the person who is promoting the "treatment" have?
4. How will the doctor evaluate your response to treatment?

These are the same questions you should be asking your surgeon, radiation therapist, and medical oncologist before starting conventional treatment.

When we're afraid and under stress, it is hard to think clearly. Facing a breast cancer diagnosis is definitely frightening and stressful. Fortunately, there are well-established methods to treat breast cancer and many options that can be tailored to an individual's preferences, beliefs, and lifestyle while still relying on evidence-based medical treatment. I encourage all women facing breast cancer to tackle fear and stress with the power of information and common sense.

When you hear that cancer can be cured in ten minutes, or that diseases as diverse as breast cancer, AIDS, and fibromyalgia can all be cured by the same herb or supplement, ask yourself, "Does that sound plausible?" Do you really want to risk your life on a product from a person you've never met, who has never examined you, and who has never seen any of the information about your specific cancer?

If you are considering or have already considered using alternative treatments alone to fight breast cancer, I strongly recommend that you also speak to experts with experience in treating breast cancer using evidence-based therapies.

CHAPTER 11

Natural Supplements
and Breast Cancer

"You have to allow yourself to feel courage,
determination, faith, hope, and love.
All nurture your will to live."
—*Andrea Gildner*

At CTCA, we have pioneered an integrative approach that combines the best of both conventional and integrative medicine. There is good clinical evidence that many patients with breast cancer benefit from an integrative approach that combines holistic treatments provided by trained experts and conventional cancer treatment. We use a variety of therapeutic approaches together with surgery, radiation, and drug treatment as part of our integrative treatment model, and all of those approaches are based on clinical evidence.

In this chapter, we will review some potential natural therapies that have been shown to provide positive impacts on quality of life during and after conventional cancer treatment.

If you want to pursue natural therapies as a part of your cancer treatment, it is important that you seek the advice of an expert with training from an accredited institution. Each naturopathic oncology provider I work with has been through four years of medical school and has been specifically trained to understand both the benefits and risks associated with the use of natural therapies. They will be the first to tell you that "natural" does not always mean "harmless." These experts can make recommendations that are unique to your body and your cancer.

Green Tea

Green tea is made from the steamed and dried leaves of the *Camellia sinesis* plant, a shrub found throughout Asia. Black tea is also made from this plant, but black tea is made from fermented leaves.

Some researchers believe that green tea may protect against certain cancers because it contains chemicals called polyphenols, which have an antioxidative effect. The most important of these appears to be a chemical called epigalocatechin (EGCG), which has been shown to prevent the development and growth of cancers in animals.

Interest in using green tea to treat or prevent breast cancer was sparked by a study published in 1998 in the *Japanese Journal of Cancer Research*. In this paper, the authors reported on 472 patients with Stages I–III breast cancer. They found that those women who drank more green tea were more likely to have breast cancer at an earlier stage and of a more favorable (hormone-sensitive) type. They also found that the women who drank more tea were less likely to see their disease recur and had longer disease-free survival.

Some other scientists have suggested that EGCG may have an effect on the HER2neu growth factor (discussed in Chapter 2). If their work is confirmed, it is possible that green tea may be of benefit when given together with conventional drug treatment to patients with Her2-positive breast cancer.

However, before we all start drinking green tea, it is important to note that a more recent study of more than fifty thousand Japanese women did not show any benefit from green tea in terms of *preventing* breast cancer. This study, published in the journal *Breast Cancer Research* in October 2010, showed no association between drinking green tea and the risk for developing breast cancer.

So, should patients with breast cancer drink green tea or not? I think we can certainly agree that there is very little risk of harm from green tea. But is there real benefit for the patient with breast cancer? In my opinion, the jury is still out on that question. More research is needed before we can say categorically that it is something we can recommend for patients with breast cancer, or for women who wish to reduce their breast cancer risk.

Vitamin D

Vitamin D is technically not a vitamin. It is the name given to a group of fat-soluble chemicals that are converted in the body into hormones (chemicals that influence body chemistry).

Vitamin D is important in a number of processes that are essential for good health, including muscle function, calcium absorption, bone formation, and normal cell division. Most people get the vitamin D they need from sunlight exposure. (When ultraviolet radiation in the sun's rays hits the skin, the skin makes more vitamin D.) Some foods contain vitamin D, including fatty fish and eggs. In the United States, some foods are *fortified* with vitamin D (meaning vitamin D is added). These include milk, fruit juices, yogurt, bread, and breakfast cereal. Your doctor can check your blood level of 25-hydoxyvitamin D with a simple blood test to make sure you're getting enough vitamin D.

There is some scientific evidence that vitamin D may play a role in reducing cancer risk, particularly the risk of bowel cancer. There have been several studies in which healthy women were given calcium and vitamin D to try to improve bone health. One study showed a 60 percent reduction in cancer incidence!

One major population study, the Third National Health and Nutrition Examination Survey, showed a major reduction in the risk of dying from colon cancer in people with higher vitamin D blood levels (the study included more than sixteen thousand people). Other studies have shown a reduction in the risk of precancerous polyps in the large bowel (colon) in patients with higher vitamin D levels.

It should be noted that a very recent study from the University of Rochester has suggested that women with *low* vitamin D levels may have an increased risk of a specific type of breast cancer, triple-negative disease, which we will discuss in Chapter 14.

Then again, many studies have failed to show any association between vitamin D levels and breast cancer risk, including the Women's Health Initiative and the National Cancer Institute's PLCO Cancer Screening Trial.

So, is there a link between vitamin D and breast cancer? Much like green tea, I believe the jury is still out. There are obvious health benefits to ensuring adequate vitamin D intake, but at this moment it doesn't appear that reduced breast cancer risk is one of them.

Before leaving the subject of vitamin D, however, I want to mention one aspect of bone health. We already discussed how postmenopausal women with ER-positive (estrogen-sensitive) breast cancer are recommended to take five years (and possibly ten years) of an aromatase inhibitor designed to reduce their body estrogen level to zero. Aromatase inhibitors increase the rate of developing osteoporosis (loss of bone protein leading to increased fracture risk). But, **a recent study of 150 women taking an aromatase inhibitor showed that adding a vitamin D supplement and calcium is successful in reducing the bone loss in these women.**

Long story short: there may well be a real advantage in taking vitamin D as part of the overall breast cancer treatment plan.

Vitamin C

Vitamin C is a water-soluble vitamin with antioxidant properties. Because of its antioxidant effect, it has been suggested as a cancer treatment for many years.

Studies in the 1970s and 1980s conducted by Linus Pauling and colleagues suggested that very large doses of vitamin C were helpful in increasing the survival time and improving the quality of life of patients with advanced cancer.

However several randomized placebo-controlled studies (of more than three hundred patients) conducted at the Mayo Clinic found no evidence of an anticancer effect due to vitamin C, and no differences in outcome between terminal patients with cancer receiving ten grams/day of vitamin C.

It was then suggested that Intravenous (IV) administration, which produces much higher blood levels of vitamin C than oral administration, might be an effective cancer treatment. Although patients can tolerate very large doses of IV vitamin C (fifty grams daily), there has been no convincing proof that these treatments help to shrink tumors or provide any sustained clinical benefit in patients with cancer.

In addition, high-dose, IV vitamin C can sometimes cause serious side effects (kidney stones, kidney failure, and possibly cataracts). It should only be administered by physicians, and its use outside of a clinical trial is not presently recommended.

Soy

Patients with breast cancer frequently ask, "Is it safe for me to eat soy products?"

Soy is widely consumed in Asia, in the form of soybeans, tofu (soybean curd), miso (fermented soybean paste), soy milk, and soy sauce. It is well recognized that Japanese women have a lower risk for developing breast cancer than American women, and that difference was often ascribed to a traditional Japanese diet, which contains a lot of soy.

Interestingly, when Japanese women emigrated to Hawaii and California and adopted a Western diet, their breast cancer numbers rose to American levels within one generation. **So what is it about soy that may protect against developing breast cancer?**

Soy contains chemicals called isoflavones, which apparently have both estrogenic and antiestrogenic activity. (If that sounds familiar, that's because it is also true of tamoxifen).

Numerous experimental and population studies, primarily in Asia, have examined soy and its possible effects on breast cancer risk. Overall it appears that a diet rich in soy, particularly during adolescence, may indeed reduce breast cancer risk, but only to a small degree.

A more important question to ask is whether patients who have breast cancer should avoid soy foods because of the possible estrogen-like effect of isoflavones. In other words, could soy actually *stimulate* the growth of breast cancer cells, and can patients with breast cancer safely eat soy foods?

There is currently no evidence of traditional soy foods (such as tofu, edamame, soy milk) stimulating the growth of breast cancer, or interfering with hormone treatment such as Tamoxifen. So I advise my patients that, based on our current knowledge, there does not appear to be any valid reason why they should avoid whole soy foods in their diets.

Bioidentical Hormones

Patients also frequently ask whether bioidentical hormones are safe. A woman enters menopause when her ovaries stop making estrogen and progesterone naturally. Loss of estrogen production will often produce a variety of symptoms including hot flashes, night sweats, depression, insomnia, loss of libido (sex drive), and vaginal dryness.

Giving estrogen and progesterone to postmenopausal women is often referred to as Hormone Replacement Therapy (HRT), and will relieve many menopausal symptoms. However, HRT is associated with increased risk of developing breast cancer, and increased risk of blood clots, heart disease, and stroke.

As a result of these findings, demonstrated in a major study called the Women's Health Initiative published in 2002, many women stopped receiving Hormone Replacement Therapy (HRT).

This reality led to the increased use of bioidentical hormones. The term refers to natural, compounded, plant-derived estrogen and progesterone. These are non-FDA approved and are generally produced by custom pharmacies. It is estimated that millions of women use bioidentical hormones. The proponents of such preparations claim that they relieve menopausal symptoms and are "natural" and therefore safe.

But, there is no scientific evidence that bioidentical hormones offer any advantage in terms of being more effective or safer than conventional FDA-approved HRT.

I am of the opinion that any woman with a history of breast cancer should not take HRT, bioidentical hormones, or any estrogen preparation. As previously discussed, a major goal of the treatment of ER-positive (estrogen-sensitive) breast cancer is to reduce estrogen effect on the breast to an absolute minimum, because estrogens stimulate the growth of ER-positive breast cancer cells.

So, for now, there is no credible scientific evidence that bioidentical hormones are safe for patients with breast cancer.

Herbs and Supplements

A survey conducted about ten years ago showed that 14 percent of all people regularly use some type of herbal medicine. Middle-aged women were the largest users of herbal medicines. In fact, 23 percent of the surveyed women in this age group had used an herbal supplement during the preceding week.

Herbs are frequently recommended for cancer prevention (1.3 million Google hits) and cancer treatment (2.5 million Google hits); however there is very limited scientific evidence from controlled clinical trials to support their use to treat cancer. Nevertheless, many patients with cancer use herbal supplements.

In the 1999 Black Women's Health Study, a group of women diagnosed with breast cancer between 1995 and 1999 were identified. Of 998 breast cancer survivors in this study, 68.2 percent had used herbal supplements, multivitamins, or both. The three most frequently used herbals were garlic (21.5 percent), gingko (12 percent), or Echinacea (9.4 percent).

There are several important points that any woman considering using herbs as part of a breast health program should be aware of:

1. Botanical preparations may be of different quality and should be obtained only from a reputable source (see also number 5 below). Be sure to consult with a trained naturopathic provider who has specific experience with cancer and works closely with oncology physicians.

2. Make sure that any preparation you take does not contain estrogens.

3. Inform all of your doctors about any and all botanical preparations you are taking. **There may be negative interactions between herbs and drugs you are prescribed.** For example, there is evidence that some herbs may interfere with or increase the effect of some chemotherapy drugs. So if you are receiving chemotherapy, your oncologist must know what botanicals you are taking. Botanicals may also interfere with anesthetics, so your surgeon must also be informed before you have surgery.

4. If you develop any symptom while taking medications that include herbs, don't assume that your herbal preparation is not the cause. Remember "natural" does not always mean "harmless."

5. Finally, please never allow an unqualified person to inject you with any substance, herbal or not. There is a real risk of contamination and serious infection from this practice.

Herbs, Menopause, and Breast Cancer

Many women use botanical preparations for the relief of menopausal symptoms, including hot flashes, weight gain, and mood changes. (We mentioned bioidentical hormones earlier in the same context.) The most common supplements used to relieve menopausal symptoms include black cohosh, red clover, soy and soy products, dong quai, evening primrose oil, ginseng, and kava.

According to the Cornell University Program on Breast Cancer and Environmental Risk Factors (BCERF), none of these herbs has consistently shown to produce a reduction in menopausal symptoms. Additionally, Cornell researchers believe several of these herbs have been shown to contain phytoestrogens (estrogen of plant origin). No good studies, however, have shown a direct causal relationship between the consumption of phytoestrogens and the development of breast cancer. Last, kava has been reported to cause serious liver damage in some patients.

So the important thing to remember is that "natural" does not always mean "harmless." Therefore, please consult trained specialists in botanical medicine, such as naturopathic providers, to determine which botanicals would be safe and beneficial in treating menopausal symptoms.

Natural Immunity

Some websites that promote alternative treatment for breast cancer claim that we are all developing cancer every day, and that a healthy immune system is constantly defending us by presumably destroying these cancers before they become clinically apparent.

If this were true, it implies that those who develop clinically obvious cancer must have a defective immune system, which can and must be improved by natural means, right? Additionally we should be able to destroy cancer by stimulating or boosting our immune system.

All scientific theories remain theories until they are proven to be correct. Is there scientific proof that immune deficiency is a cause (or *the* cause) of breast cancer? Is there proof that boosting the immune system can cure cancer?

We do have considerable experience with many thousands of patients who have defective immune systems. The most obvious examples are AIDS patients, in whom the retrovirus known as HIV (Human Immunodeficiency Virus) progressively destroys lymphocytes over many years, weakening and ultimately destroying that important component of the immune system. As a result, AIDS patient are vulnerable to many repeated infections.

Another large group of patients who have deficient immune systems are those who have received kidney, heart, or liver transplants. We give those patients antirejection drugs to deliberately weaken their immune systems so that they won't reject transplanted organs.

Now the question is: Do these patients who are undoubtedly immune suppressed have an increased incidence of cancer? The answer is YES. Patients with a weak or suppressed immune system do have an increased risk for developing cancers such as lymphoma, cancer of the cervix, Hodgkin Disease, and a previously rare skin cancer called Kaposi's Sarcoma. The common denominator among all of these cancers is that they are all linked to, and probably caused by, viral infections. It is not at all surprising that they are more common in immune-suppressed patients.

But there is no evidence of increased risk or incidence of *breast cancer* in AIDS or transplant patients.

There are also several problems with the idea of using "natural immunity therapy" to boost the body's immune system to fight cancer. The immune system is designed to fight infectious disease caused by bacteria, fungi, and viruses. The immune system is very good at recognizing foreign proteins in our bodies (meaning infections like strep, diphtheria, or polio). But if I develop cancer, that cancer is derived from *my* normal cells and contains *my* proteins. So the cancer is not "different" enough from the rest of my body to allow my immune system to recognize it as foreign and act to destroy it. That's why, with a few exceptions, immune therapy has, up until now, been of limited benefit in the treatment of patients with cancer.

Having said this, there is considerable interest among breast cancer researchers in treatments designed to use the body's own immune system to increase the effectiveness of breast cancer treatment. Studies have shown that breast cancers that have a high concentration of cancer-killing immune cells (natural killer cells) are more likely to respond well to chemotherapy. It has also been shown that certain chemotherapy drugs can increase the number of natural killer cells in a tumor, and this effect appears to be associated with a higher survival rate.

While treatments that boost the immune system are not yet ready for prime time, this is an area of active research, which may become much more widely used in the future.

My advice to all of my patients with breast cancer is this: By all means, maintain a healthy immune system through healthy diet and exercise. Such a program will help your general health and improve the quality of your life. **But it cannot in any way replace your specific cancer treatment.**

Remember: natural therapies may be very helpful in mitigating side effects of traditional cancer treatment, but they cannot cure cancer alone. If you want to pursue natural therapies as a part of your cancer treatment, be sure to seek the advice of **a specialist with a doctorate in naturopathic medicine from an accredited institution.**

CHAPTER 12

The CTCA Integrative Breast Cancer Care Model

"It was important that I didn't have to be this heroic, strong person.
I was able to concentrate on me, on getting better,
and did not have to worry about everyday things."
—*Andrea Gildner*

In the previous chapter, we described vitamins, herbs, and supplements that have been used to "treat" breast cancer. In this chapter, we will discuss the CTCA approach to cancer care that combines traditional treatment with integrative treatment to help relieve symptoms and improve the quality of life of patients undergoing treatment. The health care professionals who administer these interventions are critical members of the Breast Cancer Treatment Team at CTCA.

An Integrative Approach to Breast Cancer Care

At CTCA, our patient-centered model of care combines conventional treatment with the best of integrative therapies. We recognize that curing a patient with breast cancer requires total destruction of all visible cancer. With currently available technology, this can only be accomplished by using some combination of surgery, radiation, and drug treatments. The major goal of natural medicine in this context is *to improve quality of life* while minimizing the side effects and toxicity of cancer treatment and helping the patient maintain optimal physical, psychological, and spiritual health. As such, natural medicine and other health care professionals are important members of the CTCA health care team, and working together, we provide comprehensive care for the patient with breast cancer.

Members of the Breast Cancer Team

Modern breast cancer treatment requires a team of health care professionals with different skill sets. If you have been diagnosed with breast cancer, you will certainly need a skilled and experienced breast surgeon; a breast pathologist who has identified all of the important factors that make your cancer unique; and a medical oncologist who is familiar with the most modern and effective drug treatments for the different types of breast cancer. You will also need a radiologist to read your mammograms, breast ultrasounds, and MRIs. Depending on the specifics of your case, you might also need a radiation oncologist, a plastic (reconstructive) surgeon, and other medical specialists.

At CTCA, we believe patients also benefit from the support of a team of naturopathic oncology providers, registered dietitians, and mind-body therapists. I've listed below what I consider to be the most important qualities that everyone involved in your care should possess:

- experience with all types of breast cancer
- technical excellence in their own specialty
- broad knowledge of the medical literature relevant to breast cancer
- empathy and patience
- the opportunity, ability, and willingness to spend time and communicate with you
- the opportunity, ability, and willingness to spend time and communicate with each other
- the ability to be open minded about issues that are important to you, the patient

Basic Principles of the Integrative Cancer Care Model

1. Provide the best of conventional cancer treatment by combining the best available surgical, radiation, and drug treatments based on the individual patient's cancer type and stage, as well as other relevant health factors.

2. Improve overall quality of life by eliminating or minimizing side effects of cancer treatment.

3. Maintain optimal health and quality of life throughout cancer treatment and beyond, using the best of conventional and integrative medicine.

4. Provide appropriate support for the physical, emotional, and spiritual stress associated with cancer diagnosis and treatment.

5. Recognize the value for the patient of a team approach using the combined skills of all health care providers to develop and implement a multidisciplinary treatment program.

6. Emphasize Patient Empowerment, the concept that the patient has the right to be treated respectfully, have all of her questions answered and concerns addressed, and make her own treatment choices.

7. Provide a culture and environment in which every participant focuses on the patient and her welfare.

8. Provide an environment in which all members of the Cancer Treatment Team operate in the same facility, and communication and cross-fertilization of ideas are encouraged.

9. Recognize that a cancer diagnosis and treatment impose the need for a lifetime of observation and surveillance for cancer recurrence and long-term complications of therapy.

Naturopathic Oncology Providers

Naturopathic oncology providers at CTCA have attended one of five accredited schools of naturopathic medicine in the United States, and received a Doctor of Naturopathic Medicine (ND) degree. Currently only eighteen states license them as primary or specialty care physicians who can practice independently.

Our naturopathic oncology providers work closely with oncologists who administer conventional treatment. They prescribe natural remedies to help improve treatment effectiveness and reduce side effects. They also offer general health and emotional support and will frequently recommend natural therapies to help relieve common symptoms such as fatigue, insomnia, hot flashes, nausea and loss of appetite, pain caused by neuropathy, and joint pain.

Because long-term estrogen reduction is an important part of treatment for many patients with ER-positive breast cancer, such patients are at risk for osteoporosis later in life. Naturopathic oncology providers play an important role in helping our patients maintain good bone health, working in close cooperation with our nutrition team.

Lack of estrogen can also have major effects on a woman's libido (sex drive) and cause vaginal dryness. These, together with the loss of a breast and other major changes in body image caused by chemotherapy, can have a profound effect on a patient's relationship with her partner. It is here that compassionate and understanding care from a team of physicians, nurses, and naturopathic and mind-body professionals can be very helpful to the patient and her partner.

Registered Dietitians

It is well known that obesity, not only increases a woman's risk for developing breast cancer but also may have a negative effect on prognosis for cure. Many patients with breast cancer gain weight while receiving chemotherapy and hormone therapy—an unwelcome side effect of treatment—which may also have a negative effect on prognosis and risk of recurrence.

The advice of a registered dietitian (RD) can be very useful in helping avoid unnecessary weight gain, while ensuring the optimal intake of vitamins and minerals. The RD can also provide valuable guidance to patients whose cancer or treatment causes taste changes, lack of appetite, nausea, vomiting, diarrhea, or constipation.

A detailed discussion of dietary recommendations for the patient undergoing cancer treatment is beyond the scope of this book. Every patient receiving breast cancer treatment at CTCA, however, has the opportunity to consult regularly with her dietitian, a valued member of the Integrative Care Team.

Mind-Body Psychological Support

Many patients with cancer and their family members suffer real psychological distress, not only at the time of diagnosis but throughout their breast cancer journeys.

Our Mind-Body Team, composed of clinically trained psychotherapists and social workers, provides important support for patients and family members at times of crisis.

In addition to formal individual and group psychological counseling, many patients benefit from more symptom-oriented modalities, such as meditation, yoga, guided imagery, breathing practices, relaxation, and bodywork. Art, music, and animal-assisted therapy are all forms of mind-body support, which can greatly enhance the patient's quality of life.

I do want to mention one form of mind-body intervention that I have found very useful—and that is having a patient who is about to start breast cancer treatment meet one or two patients who have "been there, done that." It's very empowering for a woman facing chemotherapy (and the hair loss that often accompanies it) to meet a woman who went through it all two years before, has all of her own hair back, looks and feels like a million bucks, and can tell her new friend, "It's temporary. You'll get through it fine!"

I'm very grateful to my patients who volunteer their time in this way because I believe it is incredibly valuable. I'm also very thankful to groups such as Susan G. Komen for the Cure® that encourage women who have already beaten breast cancer to help and support their more recently diagnosed sisters.

Yoga

Yoga is a form of nonaerobic exercise that involves a program of precise posture, breathing exercises, and meditation. Yoga can be useful in helping the patient deal with symptoms of breast cancer and the side effects of treatment. In fact, a recent study showed that yoga could reduce side effects associated with radiation therapy.

Pastoral Care

Nurturing the spirits of patients with cancer and their families is a primary focus of our pastoral care team. Representing many faiths, they are always available to provide psychological counseling and support to those who need them.

Acupuncture

Acupuncture has been a part of traditional Chinese medicine for centuries and involves the insertion of sterile, thin needles into specific points on the skin. Controlled clinical trials have shown that acupuncture has been used successfully with patients with breast cancer to treat the nausea associated with chemotherapy and radiation and to reduce hot flashes and joint pain. Controlled clinical trials have shown improvement in patients' symptoms and overall quality of life from acupuncture treatment, with no significant adverse effects.

Always use a qualified acupuncturist, and get the OK from your doctor before you start acupuncture treatment. Whenever needles puncture the skin, there is a (small) risk of infection and bleeding, particularly if you are receiving medical treatment, such as chemotherapy or radiation, that can lower your blood counts. And if you have lymphedema (swelling of the arm on the side of your breast surgery) or are at risk for developing lymphedema, **you must not have acupuncture needles inserted in that arm** because of the risk of infection. There are alternative, noninvasive treatments your acupuncturist can use that won't increase your risk of infection.

Other Important Members of the Breast Cancer Team

Our Integrative Care Model provides much more than simply offering naturopathic medicine, nutrition, and psychological support, however. Throughout their active treatment at CTCA, our patients with breast cancer will often require the specialized services of many others in our health care team.

CTCA offers a robust integrative treatment program that involves all of the specialists listed, led by a medical oncologist responsible for working with you to find a treatment plan that will be tolerable, based on clinical recommendations and individualized to your unique cancer.

Other Important Members of the Breast Cancer Team

Chiropractic: back pain, joint mobility

Clinical Research Team: facilitate use of research techniques and drugs where appropriate

Cosmetologist: hair loss, body image issues, postmastectomy fitting

Genetic Counseling: BRCA, positive family history

Navigation: help patient and family negotiate through initial treatment planning stage

Nursing: coordination of many of the services and professionals listed in this table

Patient Representative: help patient and family negotiate through health care system

Pain Team: pain relief

Pharmacy: patient education regarding drug treatment, potential drug interactions

Physical Therapy: general conditioning, post-mastectomy frozen shoulder, post-mastectomy pain, osteoporosis, lymphedema therapy

Sexual Counseling: loss of libido, fertility issues, vaginal dryness

Social and Financial Counseling: cost of care, employment issues, disability issues

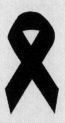

Going the Distance for Personalized Treatment

In August 1995, twenty-five-year-old Andrea Gildner felt a lump in her left breast. The 2.8-centimeter tumor—a high-grade, triple-negative cancer—was removed. Eighteen of her axillary lymph nodes tested positive for cancer. Andrea received six cycles of high-dose chemotherapy and radiation therapy to try to prevent recurrence of her disease.

In 2004, when her breast cancer recurred after nine years in remission, she was nearly ready to give up. "I had lived through chemo once and was not interested in doing it again," she explains.

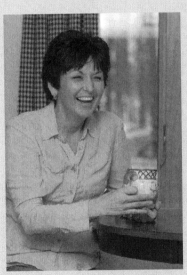

"It was important that I didn't have to be this heroic, strong person. I was able to concentrate on me, on getting better, and not have to worry about everyday things."
— Andrea Gildner

Andrea had developed an inflammatory recurrence in her left breast that left it enlarged, firm, red, and warm. Doctors performed a bilateral mastectomy. While her right breast was cancer free, the left had extensive, high-grade, triple-negative breast cancer.

After her surgery, Andrea came to CTCA and became my patient. She traveled six hundred miles for treatment, leaving her fourteen-year-old and six-year-old behind because she felt like she was out of options at home. "I never saw eye to eye with my oncologist," she told me. Her doctors back home had given her eight to twelve months to live.

The results of additional testing at CTCA did not show any evidence of metastatic or residual disease, but we knew that she was at very high risk for future recurrence.

Her tumor tested positive for a protein called EGFR, also known as HER1, a growth factor that is closely related to HER2. This knowledge helped us develop a unique treatment program for Andrea.

We used a drug called cetuximab (that specifically targets EGFR) and applied a special type of radiation called TomoTherapy® to the area of inflammatory recurrence to protect her against future disease. She remained on the cetuximab for one year and has remained free of breast cancer nine years later.

While leaving her family and young children at home was a very difficult decision for her, Andrea made many friends during her stay at CTCA. She took full advantage of our team approach and felt that the pastoral counseling and mind-body therapies were quite helpful.

"I had treatments twice a day, which wasn't fun, but one of the nice things about it was that I was allowed to face my fears," Andrea says. "At home, I had to keep a strong face for my kids, my husband, and my parents. I couldn't break down. At CTCA, I could break down, go to group therapy, and talk about it openly. I didn't have to prepare meals, go through my kids' book bags, or otherwise wear all the hats I had to wear at home. It was important that I didn't have to be this heroic, strong person. I was able to concentrate on me, on getting better, and [did] not have to worry about everyday things.

"You have to take charge and look for options for treatment," Andrea concludes. "This needs to be just about you! Cancer was never a chapter that I wanted in my book. But I wouldn't trade all I've learned because of this experience."

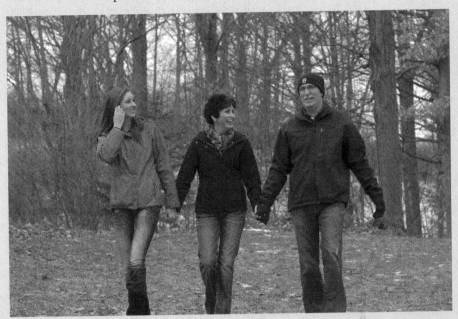

Doctor's Comments

Andrea's story teaches us that no two patients or tumors are identical. In the modern era of personalized cancer care, the more we learn about the genetic makeup of the cancer, the more treatment can be tailored to the specifics of the disease and the individual patient.

Targeted treatments are more specific, and therefore less toxic and more effective. In 1995, Andrea was initially given a 3 percent chance of survival. As of June 2013, Andrea remains in good health, with no evidence of recurrent breast cancer.

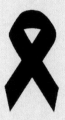

Fighting Silent Cancers

DIANE BUTLER-HUGHES'S BREAST CANCER JOURNEY began in 1998 when she was thirty-eight years old. That's when she noticed a thickening of her right breast. Her OB/GYN said, "We can't get biopsies for everyone who finds a lump." But that doctor should most definitely have known better, since Diane's aunt and cousin both had breast cancer.

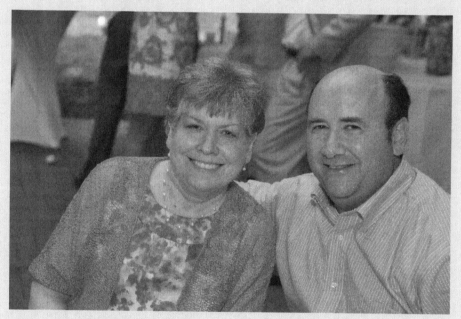

"It's amazing what women with cancer can accomplish!"
— *Diane Butler-Hughes, with her husband David*

Diane had a negative mammogram, which reinforced the doctor's idea that a biopsy was unnecessary. In the meantime, Diane could feel something growing. She finally went to see a surgeon, one week after getting married. The meeting did not go well. The surgeon did not have a good bedside manner, and Diane didn't understand what was being recommended to her or why.

In the end, another surgeon performed nine core biopsies, all of which came back positive. In May 2000, two weeks before her forty-first birthday, Diane was diagnosed with Stage III, ER-positive, PR-positive, invasive lobular breast cancer.

Lobular cancer is often difficult to detect on a mammogram, which is why Diane's mammogram, completed only two weeks before her diagnosis, was reported as normal. Thirteen of her twenty-six axillary nodes on the right side were positive for cancer. Two months later, she had a mastectomy and reconstruction. The mass removed was eight centimeters in diameter.

After surgery, Diane received chemotherapy, radiation, and appropriate hormone treatment.

Diane remained apparently cancer free for four years. Throughout this process, she did lots of research and became a strong, well-informed advocate for herself. At her request, her doctor ordered a bone scan and CAT scan every year, and nearly five years later, a bone scan showed a spot on her spine.

In 2004, she came to CTCA upon the advice of a friend. In the months that followed, she had laparoscopic surgery to remove her ovaries (oophorectomy) and was switched from tamoxifen to another estrogen blocker called anastrazole. She also began taking a monthly injection of zoledronic acid, a bone-protective drug we use to help prevent bone destruction by metastatic cancer cells. Radiation therapy to her lumbar spine and ongoing systemic treatment held the disease more or less in check for a few years.

In April 2007, measurements of a substance produced by cancer cells called carcinoembryonic antigen (CEA), used to monitor the effectiveness of treatment, showed rising levels, at which point we switched Diane's anastrazole for another drug, letrozole, which belongs to the same drug class. When her CEA levels rose again in March 2008, a PET scan showed progression of the metastases in her bones, but no metastases to her organs.

Since then, Diane has been on several drugs to keep the cancer under control. At the time of this writing in July 2013, Diane is once again in an excellent remission while taking a very effective combination of pills (everolimus and exemestane).

Diane is now an advocate for other women with breast cancer. She tells her story in council meetings and churches and was instrumental in having the Smoke Free Ohio Workplace legislation passed in Ohio in 2006. Having worked in the restaurant industry for seventeen years, she remains convinced that exposure to secondhand smoke had an effect on her body.

Diane is a strong believer in naturopathic medicine and nutrition and relied on these specialists at CTCA throughout her treatment. "My naturopathic oncology provider is just as important to me as my oncologist," she says. "I've learned so much from my naturopathic providers. They've helped with supplements to boost my immune system, minimize side effects, and help with neuropathy."

In 2003, Diane and seven other cancer survivors founded a nonprofit organization called the Noble Circle Project. They provide retreats and classes that focus on complementary energy techniques, nutritional education, and peer support and have served nearly 200 women to date. "It's amazing what women with cancer can accomplish!" she says.

Doctor's Comments

Lobular carcinoma of the breast can be difficult to diagnose. Both clinical findings and the mammogram often show very little abnormality, so doctors have to have a low threshold for ordering a biopsy. Diane's case provides an example of how patients with lobular carcinoma often have more advanced disease at the time of diagnosis.

Despite presenting with Stage III disease more than twelve years ago and relapsing with bone involvement nearly five years later, Diane still maintains an excellent quality of life. Lobular carcinoma frequently involves bone, and because it is frequently ER-positive, will often respond to hormone treatment.

Diane also benefited from palliative radiation to the lumbar spine early on, and her experience also demonstrates the value of bone protective agents given together with chemotherapy and hormone therapy to prevent serious complications from the tumors in her bone, such as fracture and high blood calcium.

Finally, she has enjoyed excellent quality of life for nearly eight years, while her disease has been held in check by a series of different drug treatments. Throughout that time she has benefited greatly from many of the supportive health programs provided by our Breast Cancer Treatment Team.

CHAPTER 13

Metastatic Breast Cancer Is Not a Hopeless Situation

"I was basically given a death sentence and I thought, 'I am not accepting this.'"
—*Rosalind Landrum*

At the present time, patients with metastatic breast cancer cannot be totally cured of their disease, but there is plenty of room for cautious optimism when faced with this diagnosis.

First a word about *cure*. Cure means killing every cancer cell in the body that we can identify, such that no additional or maintenance treatment is needed. When treatment is completed, the patient who is cured has no sign of cancer, doesn't need any more treatment, and has the same life expectancy as someone of similar age who never had cancer.

It is certainly true that many thousands of patients with cancers like leukemia, lymphoma, Hodgkin Disease, testicular cancer, and many childhood cancers have been cured of advanced cancer. Although their stories are an inspiration for everyone, their experience is not really relevant to women with metastatic breast cancer. Why not?

The cancers referred to above are all characterized by being extremely sensitive to radiation and chemotherapy. They frequently just melt away with appropriate treatment. So we confidently expect that most patients with these types of cancer will be completely cured. But that's not yet true for most solid tumors in adults with cancers of the colon, lung, ovary, bladder, and breast.

In this chapter, we discuss in detail how medical oncologists approach the patient with Stage IV breast cancer. Before doing so, however, I want to make an important point that contains a message of real hope.

Over the past forty years, we have seen major advances in how effective our treatments are for Stage IV breast cancer. All the time you read about "The Cure" for cancer. Well that's kind of a simplistic view, in my opinion.

Rather than a single, earth-shattering announcement of "The Cure," what we have seen are small sequential steps. These represent many advances in our knowledge of the science of breast cancer, resulting in improved treatment.

Take a look at the table which shows one institution's experience in how treatments have improved over a twenty-five-year period.

	Median Survival (range)	5 Year Survival
1974–1979	15 months (11–19)	10%
1990–1994	27 months (21–33)	29%
1995–2000	51 months (33–69)	40%

Stage IV breast cancer is a *highly* treatable condition.

There are now a large number of drugs available that are highly active against breast cancer and will frequently produce significant clinical remissions in patients with advanced disease. We discussed the different classes of agents that are available in Chapter 6.

In general, it is the biologic nature of the cancer that directs the medical oncologist to choose an appropriate treatment program. ER-positive cancers are frequently well controlled by hormone therapy, and HER2neu-positive cancers are best treated by drugs like trastuzumab and lapatinib—drugs that specifically target the HER2neu pathway. These are examples of treatment that *target* specific proteins present in some breast cancers.

General Approach to the Patient with Metastatic Breast Cancer (Stage IV Disease)

1. Stage IV breast cancer is a *highly* treatable condition.
2. Most patients with metastatic breast cancer cannot be totally cured.
3. No two patients with metastatic breast cancer are identical.
4. There is a degree of uncertainty with every treatment.
5. When patients respond to drug treatment, it frequently opens up other treatment options.

In contrast with targeted therapy, most chemotherapy drugs are much less specific in their action. They are more generally cytotoxic, meaning they have the potential to kill all living cells.

Generally, cancer cells are more susceptible to being killed by chemotherapy than healthy cells, although it is damage to healthy cells that leads to chemotherapy side effects (such as hair loss, fatigue, and low blood counts).

There are no very good predictive tests that will tell your doctor with absolute certainty which of the numerous chemotherapy drugs available is the right one for your cancer.

Most patients with metastatic breast cancer cannot be totally cured.

If we cannot realistically destroy every single cancer cell, such that total cure is feasible, what can we do? As you recall, there are several reasons why we treat patients with Stage IV breast cancer:

1. To improve the patient's quality of life by relieving symptoms caused by the cancer
2. To prolong disease-free and symptom-free survival
3. To prevent and to treat complications of the cancer
4. To relieve distress and support the patient and family throughout her illness

The modern approach to the patient with metastatic breast cancer is to change it into a chronic illness that the patient can live with *for years*.

When explaining this to patients, I use the following example: Patients with chronic illnesses such as high blood pressure, diabetes, or rheumatoid arthritis give themselves shots or take pills every day to *control* their disease. These patients are not *cured*. They are living with a chronic illness, but it will not cause major symptoms or seriously interfere with their lives, as long as they take their medication regularly. And that's the modern approach to advanced breast cancer.

No two patients with metastatic breast cancer are identical.

There are many factors specific to the type of breast cancer, and the individual patient that must be considered when evaluating every patient with metastatic breast cancer. The experienced medical oncologist recognizes this and adjusts the treatment he or she recommends to reflect this.

The following is a chart of factors that we use to determine the prognosis for every patient with recurrent breast cancer. We will discuss several of these in some detail.

Prognostic Factors in the Patient with Recurrent Breast Cancer

	FAVORABLE	UNFAVORABLE
Disease-free interval:	long	short
Organs involved:	skin, lymph node, bone	brain, liver, lung
Number of sites involved:	few	many
Estrogen-Receptor status:	positive	negative
Comorbidities:	absent	present
Serious organ dysfunction:	absent	present
Performance status:	0–1	3–4
Number of previous drug treatments:	few	many
Circulating tumor cells	0–5	>5

Disease-Free Interval

Most patients with breast cancer have early stage disease (Stage 0, I, or II) at the time of first diagnosis. Only about 5 percent (one in twenty) has metastatic (Stage IV) disease at the time of first diagnosis.

As a result, most people are treated initially for early stage disease. And for many thousands of women, that treatment is successful, and their cancers never recur. They are cured of breast cancer, and they have the same life expectancy as any other woman of the same age.

But in about 30 percent of women with apparently early disease, the disease comes back, either in the general area of the breast (including chest wall and armpit) or at a more distant site, such as the liver, bone, or lung.

In such patients, we measure the disease-free interval defined as the time from first diagnosis and treatment until the first recurrence of disease. This is an important factor that provides a lot of information about the biologic nature of the cancer and the aggressiveness of its growth.

Think of it this way: if it takes only a few *months* for a cancer to show up again after surgery removed all of the apparent disease, then that's a much more aggressive cancer than one that takes *years* to reappear. The shorter the disease-free interval, the more aggressive the cancer and the more aggressive the treatment needs to be to get it under control.

Organs Involved

Broadly speaking, recurrent breast cancer that involves the skin of the chest wall, lymph nodes in the axilla, the neck, or bone tend to be easier to treat and less serious than metastases involving liver, lung, or other internal organs.

Metastases in the brain pose a special problem for several reasons. As the brain is enclosed in the skull, a rigid structure that cannot stretch to accommodate a growing mass, brain metastases often produce a rise in pressure within the skull, and this can have serious consequences.

Furthermore, most anticancer drugs don't cross from the blood into the brain, so chemotherapy that may be very effective against advanced cancer elsewhere in the body often won't help against brain metastases. (That's why we usually use radiation for brain tumors.)

In addition to the *specific* organs affected, the *number* of metastatic sites is also important. As you would expect, it is better to have one or two areas of metastatic disease rather than dozens. Like disease-free interval, the overall *tumor load* speaks to the biologic aggressiveness of the cancer and how quickly the cancer is likely to be life threatening for the patient.

Estrogen-Receptor Status (ER)

ER-positive breast cancers tend to grow more slowly than ER-negative tumors. Additionally, we have a powerful weapon—hormone therapy—that we can use when treating patients with ER-positive disease.

Comorbidities, Organ Dysfunction, Performance Status, and Number of Prior Therapies

By comorbidities, we mean diseases other than cancer. It is much easier to treat a patient who is generally healthy than one who is very sick. If the patient has other serious medical conditions, such as heart failure or serious liver or kidney disease, it will be much more difficult for the oncologist to treat her with the intensity needed to control her cancer.

Many of our chemotherapy drugs are excreted from the body by the kidney, or are detoxified by the liver, so it is important that these organs are working well for the best possible results from treatment.

That is not to say that we can't treat a patient if she's on regular dialysis for kidney failure, for example. We have done it many times, but it certainly adds a degree of complexity to the treatment plan.

Performance status is a measure of how *active* the patient is. Broadly speaking, treatment is more likely to be effective and better tolerated in the patient if the cancer has not caused her to become severely restricted in her activities (or worse, bedridden).

When treating patients with advanced breast cancer, we are fortunate to have a large number of very active drugs available. If a patient has received only one or two prior drug treatments, then more treatment options will be available.

* * *

A rational treatment plan is developed for a patient based on all of these factors, in addition to the important biologic variables of the tumor. Please remember that these are *general rules* only; there are always exceptions to any rules.

There is a degree of uncertainty with every medical treatment of metastatic breast cancer.

If a patient has strep throat, she can be pretty sure that penicillin will cure her. The diabetic patient can be fairly confident that insulin will control her diabetes. In contrast, there is a degree of uncertainty whenever a medical oncologist treats a patient with advanced cancer with a new drug. There are no good predictive tests that can reliably tell in advance if a cancer is sensitive to a particular chemotherapy drug. That's just the limitation of the science of oncology at this time.

Your doctor will certainly know from his/her prior experience and the published literature that a certain drug has produced significant benefits in patients with advanced breast cancer. But there is no guarantee that it will be beneficial in the treatment of *your* cancer. So the only way to find out is to give you the drug and observe the effect.

I mention this because I frequently see patients who have been given a dire prognosis from their doctors, *even before they have received any treatment*. This doesn't make any sense. No one really knows whether the patient will respond to future treatment, and if they do, for how long. It is unfair to any patient who is starting what may be a long and difficult journey to "tell" her what the end result will be, especially as the doctor really has no idea what the future holds for her.

The most appropriate approach is to adopt a cautiously optimistic attitude. We do not encourage unrealistic hope, but neither should we overemphasize the negative.

Positive Response to Drug Treatment Opens Other Treatment Options

When patients respond to drug treatment with shrinkage or total disappearance of their tumors, it often opens up other treatment options, which can include surgery or radiation. In this book you will read about several patients who directly benefited from this approach.

Before we leave the subject of metastatic breast cancer, I want to emphasize that this an area of constant research, aimed at increasing our knowledge and improving treatment options. The more we learn about the biology of breast cancer and the specific cellular targets that breast cancer cells often contain, the more rational, specific, and effective our treatments will become.

Modern oncology offers many treatment options that can produce meaningful remissions, often measured in years. And throughout her life with advanced cancer, the patient and her family will benefit from kindness, honesty, and optimism from her doctors, in addition to the best that medical science can offer.

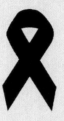

Stage IV With A Future

ROSALIND LANDRUM DEVELOPED CANCER of the left breast in 2000 at the age of fifty-one. There were three distinct tumors in the breast, and the largest was 1.5 centimeters. Rosalind underwent a left mastectomy and axillary node dissection. The pathology results showed that three nodes were positive, and the tumor was ER strongly positive and HER2 negative.

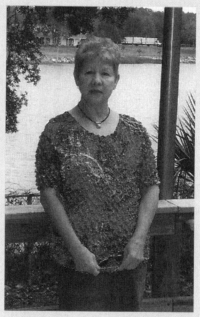

"Take each fear one at a time and know that there is
something inside of you that is bigger than all of your fears."
— Rosalind Landrum

Rosalind had immediate breast reconstruction, followed by chemotherapy and postmastectomy radiation. She then began taking adjuvant tamoxifen.

Four years later, she discovered the cancer had spread to her liver, lungs, and bones. Her doctor was less than encouraging. "I was basically given a death sentence," she says, "and I thought, 'I am not accepting this.'" In December 2004, Rosalind came to CTCA for the first time.

"When I arrived at CTCA, I asked, 'Is there hope?' Dr. Citrin said, 'There is always hope.' In that moment, my whole life changed," Rosalind says.

At CTCA, Rosalind received six cycles of chemotherapy with docetaxel and carboplatin every three weeks and experienced an excellent reduction in tumor masses. During the summer of 2005, she received a special type of radiation called TomoTherapy® to the residual disease in her liver. Following radiation, Rosalind was then started on maintenance exemestane, which she continues to the present date (October 2013).

Currently she is in a complete remission with no symptoms, has normal physical examination and normal tumor markers, zero circulating tumor cells visible in her blood, and entirely normal scans.

Today, Rosalind is enjoying life with her husband, son, and ten-year-old granddaughter. She advises women to trust their doctors and be confident that they care about you. She also says, "One of the main fears of going through cancer are all of the unknowns. Take each fear one at a time and know that there is something inside of you that is bigger than all of your fears. Stay positive! Turn negative talk into something positive! And believe in the miracles from our Lord."

Doctor's Comments

Rosalind's story is very inspiring and teaches us several important lessons. She came to us with very advanced metastatic disease occupying more than half of her liver. Despite her local doctor's dire prognosis, Rosalind is in a complete remission from her cancer eight years later.

Her story (and that of countless other patients with similar stories) demonstrate why doctors should never give a prognosis to a patient, even if they have advanced disease, until they (the doctors) have treated the patient and observed the effects of that treatment.

But Rosalind's experience teaches us a lot more. First, when patients like Rosalind respond well to chemotherapy treatment, it often opens up many more treatment options.

Rosalind also demonstrates the value of the multidisciplinary approach that we advocate at CTCA. Radiation therapy is generally ineffective against liver metastases because of the relatively low radiation tolerance of normal liver tissue. But by using the elegant technique of TomoTherapy® to maximize radiation to the few cancerous areas that remained after chemotherapy, we were able to effectively kill the cancers in her liver, while sparing healthy liver tissue.

Finally, after undergoing an arduous treatment program of chemotherapy and radiation, which resulted in a complete remission, Rosalind has benefited from simple hormone therapy to maintain that remission for nearly eight years.

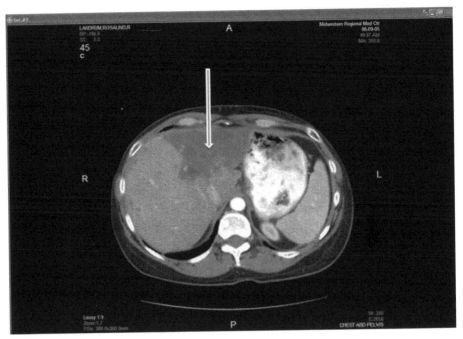

CAT scan of Rosalind Landrum's upper abdomen shows a massive tumor involving the left lobe of liver. Taken in June 2005.

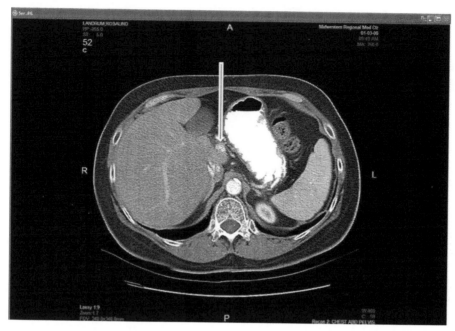

This follow-up CAT scan (taken in January 2008) shows that the massive tumor has been eradicated. A tiny area of calcification can be seen in the left lobe of the liver. There is no evidence of residual cancer. Most recent studies remain entirely normal.

CHAPTER 14

Special Clinical Situations

Throughout this book, I have tried to emphasize that no two patients are identical, and that the modern approach to breast cancer care is to *personalize* treatment to fit the individual patient and her cancer. Within that general idea, however, is the recognition that some patients have a breast cancer which presents special challenges. Some of these special clinical situations are discussed in this chapter:

Inflammatory Breast Cancer
Triple-Negative Breast Cancer
BRCA
Breast Cancer in African American Women
Breast Cancer in Young Women
The Contralateral (opposite) Breast
Breast Cancer During Pregnancy and the Lactating Breast
Breast Cancer after Hodgkin Disease
Invasive Lobular Carcinoma
Lobular Carcinoma in Situ
Breast Cancer in Men
Paget's Disease
Brain Metastasis
Bone Metastasis

Inflammatory Breast Cancer

Long before antibiotics were developed, many women developed bacterial infections in the breast. This was particularly common among women who were nursing, but the problem could occur at any time.

Infections in the breast are no different from infections anywhere else in the body. They produce *inflammation* of the skin, which is recognized by the presence of pain and tenderness, redness, swelling, and increased warmth.

For more than a century, we have known that when some women showed all the signs of inflammation in one breast, the cause might not be infection but in fact a special type of breast cancer known as inflammatory breast cancer.

What characterizes inflammatory breast cancer is early invasion of the skin of the breast by cancer cells, resulting in an inflamed appearance to the breast. Inflammatory breast cancer accounts for only 1 percent to 2 percent of all invasive breast cancers. It tends to occur in younger women, and its treatment is different from other forms of breast cancer.

Inflammatory breast cancer represents a very rapidly growing cancer that invades blood vessels and lymphatic channels very early. It has often spread to lymph nodes, lung, or liver by the time it is diagnosed. It is important to note that **there is frequently no definite lump palpable in the breast**. Rather, there is just a heaviness or general swelling of all or part of the affected breast.

Because the disease is relatively rare and the clinical findings are unusual, it is common for the diagnosis to be delayed, often for a month or two, while the patient is treated with several courses of antibiotics (which are of no benefit, of course).

Any woman with a breast that looks like this and has had two weeks of antibiotics with no resolution of the situation should insist on consulting a breast specialist. She needs an urgent biopsy, not of the breast tissue alone but also of the affected *skin*.

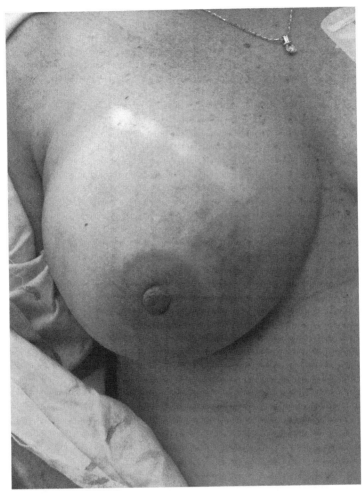

Typical appearance of early inflammatory breast cancer with a skin rash. Note also that the nipple is partially obscured by the edema (swelling) of the breast.

Inflammatory breast cancer has a very bad reputation. Because of the skin involvement, many patients who were previously treated with mastectomy very quickly developed tumor recurrence in the mastectomy scar. I've seen such recurrence within a few *weeks* of mastectomy.

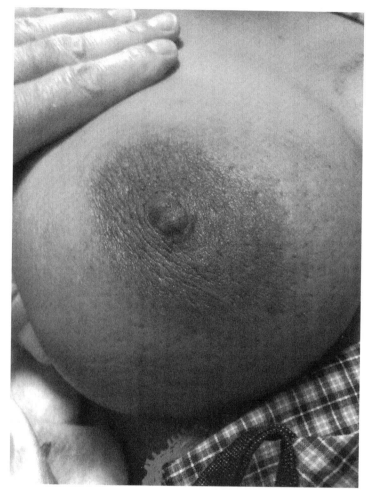

Inflammatory breast cancer in an African-American patient with swelling of the entire lower breast and an orange peel appearance.

Because we now recognize the special nature of inflammatory breast cancer, modern, multidisciplinary treatment that includes high-dose chemotherapy as the first line of treatment has fundamentally changed the course of this disease for many women. Regardless of its bad reputation, inflammatory breast cancer can no longer be considered a hopeless situation.

There is no question that effective treatment of any patient with inflammatory breast cancer—one that includes an optimal use of drug treatment, surgery, and radiation—requires a cooperative effort from all members of the health care team. For that reason, I strongly recommend that every woman with inflammatory breast cancer receive treatment from a team of physicians with special expertise in this challenging condition.

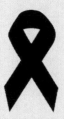

Inflammatory Breast Cancer Is Highly Treatable

TERI WENTWORTH FIRST NOTICED REDNESS ON THE SKIN of the underside of her right breast in 2010. She was fifty-seven at the time. The photos she found on the Internet didn't look like what she saw on her own breast, so she didn't immediately seek medical help.

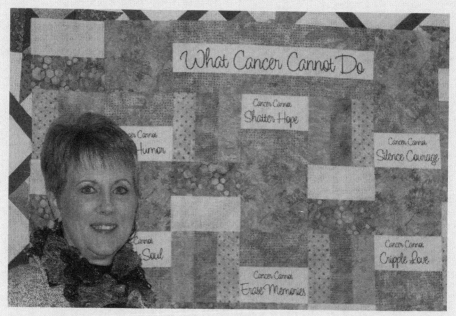

"Once you find a doctor you trust, do whatever he tells you to do."
— *Teri Wentworth*

A mammogram revealed abnormal areas in the breast that were quite different from what appeared on her last mammogram three years earlier, and the biopsy that followed led to a diagnosis of invasive ductal cell cancer. She was told it was very treatable. In her conversation with the surgeon, who was not a specialist in breast cancer surgery, he told her that she needed a mastectomy, but that it "wasn't rocket science."

Teri's two brothers encouraged her to seek a second opinion, and Teri came to CTCA to be evaluated. It was immediately clear to us that Teri had inflammatory breast cancer, a cancer that should not be treated initially with a mastectomy.

My examination of her breast detected an additional two-centimeter mass, and a biopsy confirmed invasive, high-grade ductal carcinoma that was ER/PR negative and HER2neu positive. The disease had already spread throughout the breast, chest wall, and axillary nodes. A CAT scan found lung and liver metastases.

Teri's presentation was typical of inflammatory breast cancer, with rapid development of breast symptoms and the presence of distant metastases at the time of first diagnosis. When I first saw her, her right breast was enlarged, heavy, and red. After eight cycles of chemotherapy with docetaxel, carboplatin, and trastuzumab, she achieved complete remission. She had no sickness at all from the chemo but says, "Things just tasted funny."

"Get checked as soon as you know something's up," Teri advises others. "Don't let it go. Be sure to get a second opinion. And once you find a doctor you trust, do whatever he [or she] tells you to do."

We started Teri's treatment in April 2010, and at this writing in January 2014, she remains very well. She comes to CTCA once every three weeks for IV-maintenance therapy. She is fully active and has no evidence of active disease.

Teri is being maintained in a complete remission on HER2-directed therapy alone and is living entirely free of symptoms.

Doctor's Comments

Teri's story is a classic example of inflammatory breast cancer, with rapid development of breast symptoms and distant metastases at the time of first diagnosis. You'll note that it had been almost three years since her last screening mammogram.

Inflammatory breast cancer historically has a bad reputation, but even this disease can no longer be considered a hopeless situation. Modern, multidisciplinary treatment—the foundation of which is initial high-dose chemotherapy—has fundamentally changed the course of this disease for many women.

Teri's experience demonstrates the tremendous advances in treatment that result from accurate identification of the molecular subtype of the cancer.

Another important lesson from Teri's story is that women should seek the advice of breast care specialists in medical oncology, surgery, and radiation. The first doctor she saw recommended immediate mastectomy, yet all experts in the field of breast cancer agree that surgery is not the first recommended treatment for inflammatory breast cancer.

Triple-Negative Breast Cancer

Many breast cancers contain one or more of the specialized proteins ER, PR, and HER2neu, and we have already discussed how these proteins (particularly ER and HER2neu) represent useful *targets* for treatment.

Hormone therapy, which targets the estrogen receptor, is very effective treatment for ER-positive breast cancer, while treatments such as trastuzumab and lapatinib that specifically target HER2neu are very effective for HER2-positive breast cancer.

In contrast, *triple-negative* breast cancers do not contain ER, PR, or HER2neu proteins and do not have specific cellular targets that we can attack. In 2008, it was estimated that more than one million women were diagnosed worldwide with breast cancer and that more than one hundred seventy thousand were classified as having triple-negative disease.

Although triple-negative breast cancer can occur in any woman, it is found most frequently in three specific groups: very young women (less than forty years of age), African-American women, and women with BRCA1-gene mutation.

We now know that there is no single-entity, triple-negative breast cancer. Molecular subtyping has identified four or five major subtypes. There is a great deal of active research in this area, and it is likely that specific targeted treatments will be developed for each subtype.

Here are a few important points to emphasize about triple-negative disease:

1. It is a relatively fast-growing cancer.
2. Cure rates are not as high as other breast cancers of similar stage.
3. It tends to recur within one to three years of initial diagnosis.
4. There is a relatively high risk of the disease spreading to the brain.
5. It is not responsive to hormone-blocking or HER2neu-directed treatment.

But the news is not all bad with regard to triple-negative breast cancer. Because it is a rapidly growing disease, triple-negative breast cancer appears to be very sensitive to chemotherapy drugs, specifically cisplatin, carboplatin, gemcitabine, and possibly also a new class of drugs, PARP inhibitors. (See BRCA below.)

Recall Jennifer Barber's story from the introduction to this book? Jennifer felt a lump in her breast but was so fearful that she didn't seek medical treatment for six months. Jennifer's tumor was triple negative, and during that six-month delay, the cancer grew much bigger and spread to the armpit nodes. By the time she came to see me, her tumor was very large, as you can see in the MRI image on page 115.

But triple-negative cancers are frequently highly sensitive to chemotherapy, and Jennifer's tumor proved to be no exception. After four chemotherapy treatments, the massive tumor in her breast and armpit lymph nodes had shrunk so much that Jennifer was able to have limited (breast-conserving) surgery.

All of the residual abnormality that can be seen on the repeat MRI image was only scar tissue. At the time of surgery, there was no microscopic evidence of residual cancer cells. So Jennifer's prognosis for a complete cure is excellent.

While this is a very encouraging result for Jennifer, there is no question that triple-negative breast cancer presents a formidable challenge for many women. Just like inflammatory breast cancer, I recommend that any woman who has been diagnosed with triple-negative breast cancer receive treatment from a team of physicians with special expertise in this challenging condition.

BRCA and Other Hereditary Cancers

It has been known for many years that if a woman has a positive family history for breast cancer, then she has a greater than average risk of developing the disease.

In 1988, a specific gene abnormality, known as a *mutation,* was identified as being responsible for an inherited susceptibility for developing breast cancer.

It is now known that there are two major gene mutations—known as BRCA1 and BRCA2—that increase a woman's risk for developing breast cancer and ovarian cancer.

Mutations in BRCA1 and BRCA2 account for 80 percent to 90 percent of cases of hereditary breast cancer. There are other, less common gene mutations unrelated to BRCA, which also significantly increase the risk of developing breast cancer. These include P53 and PTEN. Mutations in P53 greatly increase the risk for developing many cancers, with a 90 percent risk of cancer by age fifty. Breast cancer is the most common cancer seen in women with the P53 mutation. Approximately 80 percent of women with PTEN mutation will develop breast cancer by age seventy.

What all of these genes have in common is that they are responsible for the repair of damaged cells. Known as *tumor-suppressor genes,* they function to prevent cells that have been damaged by various environmental factors from becoming cancer cells. Changes or mutations in these genes make their tumor-suppressive function ineffective, resulting in an increased risk for developing cancer.

There are other gene mutations that are less common in most populations and are likely to increase a woman's chances of developing breast cancer, although to far lesser extent than BRCA.

My advice to any woman who has several family members with breast cancer is to seek the advice of a genetic counselor.

BRCA

As BRCA mutations are the most common gene mutations associated with increased breast cancer risk, we'll discuss them in more detail.

BRCA Mutation and Cancer Risk

- Increased lifetime risk for breast cancer

- Breast cancer at young age

- Risk of second cancer in opposite breast

- BRCA1 associated with triple negative cancer

- Higher risk for cancer of ovary, prostate cancer (in men), and other cancers (pancreas)

- More intensive screening is appropriate.

- Prophylactic bilateral mastectomy and removal of ovaries and tubes should be considered.

- Other risk-reducing treatments include tamoxifen.

- PARP inhibitors may be very effective drug treatment.

Mutations of BRCA are rare in most populations, occurring in approximately one in four hundred people, but they are much more common in people of Eastern European origin (Ashkenazic Jews), in which one in forty people carries one of three main mutations—so-called founder mutations.

Although BRCA mutations are most commonly seen in people of Eastern European Jewish descent, they are by no means exclusive to that population.

A recent study in the San Francisco Bay area reported the following incidence of BRCA1 mutations in different ethnic groups: 3.5 percent Hispanics, 1.3 percent Asian Americans, 8.3 percent Ashkenazic Jews, and 2.2 percent non-Hispanic whites.

Because the BRCA gene is not carried on the sex chromosome, BRCA mutations can affect men, and men with such a mutation have an increased risk for developing breast cancer (see the section on male breast cancer later in this chapter).

Women with mutations in BRCA1 have a lifetime risk of developing breast cancer in the range of 50 percent to 80 percent, while the risk for a woman with BRCA2 mutation is approximately 40 percent to 70 percent. Lifetime risk of cancer of the ovary is approximately 40 percent for women with BRCA1 and 20 percent for BRCA2 mutations.

It's important to mention that not only is the risk of breast cancer much higher, but also the age of onset of the disease is frequently much younger.

The type of breast cancer seen in women with BRCA1 mutations is frequently triple negative, as we discussed earlier in this chapter. The cancer seen in women with BRCA2 mutations are less commonly triple negative and are more similar to that seen in the general population.

Before leaving BRCA, I want to make several additional points. The risk of a second cancer developing at a later date in the opposite breast is significant (approximately 3 percent of patients will develop cancer in the opposite breast every year).

Women with BRCA mutations need earlier and more intensive screening for cancer of the breast and ovary, with screening mammograms and breast MRI, beginning at age twenty-five.

We will discuss bilateral prophylactic mastectomy (surgical removal of both breasts to prevent the development of breast cancer) below. Because the risk of cancer of the ovary is significant, removal of both ovaries at age thirty-five to forty is often recommended in women with a BRCA mutation. An additional advantage of removal of the ovaries is that by itself, it significantly reduces the risk of developing breast cancer.

Finally, it's not all bad news. Breast cancer in BRCA-positive patients appears to be highly sensitive to a new and exciting class of drugs known as PARP inhibitors. There is currently a great deal of active research in this area, and it is likely that PARP inhibitors will play an increasingly important role in the treatment of breast (and ovarian) cancer in BRCA-positive patients in the future.

Suspected Hereditary Cancer

So what should a person do if she suspects she has an increased genetic risk for developing breast cancer? It's important to know that a simple blood test will tell you with a high degree of confidence whether you have a significant gene mutation or not. Such information is highly confidential and cannot be used to discriminate against you in terms of employment, health, or life insurance.

If any of the situations shown in the table apply to you or your family, I strongly recommend that you consult a genetic counselor, a health care professional specially trained in genetics.

The genetic counselor will create a detailed genetic history, and help you understand exactly what is your risk for developing cancer of the breast, and other diseases. The genetic counselor is an important member of our Breast Cancer Team.

When to Consider Genetic Testing

You should seek professional genetic counseling if you or any family member has any of the following:

- known gene mutation in the family
- patient or close relative diagnosed with breast cancer before age forty-five, especially if multiple cases of breast cancer
- a high rate of bilateral breast cancers
- any male relative with breast cancer
- patient or close relative diagnosed with cancer of ovary or fallopian tube
- multiple family members with cancer of the pancreas (especially if Eastern European Jewish)

Bilateral Prophylactic Mastectomy

We've already discussed the very real lifetime risk for developing breast cancer in women with a documented mutation in BRCA, or other less common gene mutation.

Surgically removing both breasts in a healthy woman when she has no sign of breast cancer seems like a very radical recommendation. So what's the evidence to support such a recommendation?

There are numerous studies that show that surgical removal of both breasts in women with a BRCA mutation reduces her risk of developing breast cancer by approximately 95 percent. Women in these studies who chose not to have prophylactic mastectomy were significantly more likely to develop breast cancer during follow up.

For women who choose bilateral mastectomy, there are different surgical techniques available, including nipple-sparing and subcutaneous mastectomies, and many different methods for breast reconstruction.

I advise any woman contemplating prophylactic mastectomy to consult with all of the relevant medical specialists: breast surgeon, plastic surgeon, breast oncologist, and genetics specialist before making a decision.

Breast Cancer in African-American Women

Breast cancer is the most commonly diagnosed cancer among African-American women. An estimated 27,060 new cases of breast cancer are expected to occur among African-American women in 2013. Among younger women (under age forty-five), the mortality rate of breast cancer has been reported to be higher in African Americans than in whites.

African-American women develop breast cancer at a younger age than white women and are more likely to have disease of a higher grade and more advanced stage.

Younger African-American women in particular appear to have a higher risk for triple-negative breast cancers, which we discussed earlier in this chapter. The reason for this is unclear but may be related to certain reproductive patterns that are more common among African-American women (including giving birth to more than one child, a younger age at their first period, and early age at first pregnancy) and may be associated with increased risk of aggressive subtypes of breast cancer. It is clear that young African-American women with aggressive breast cancer require vigorous drug treatment.

A recent study of triple-negative breast cancer from the MD Anderson Cancer Center in Houston showed that African-American women who achieve an excellent result from such chemotherapy have as good a prognosis as women of other races.

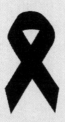

Special Care with African-American Women

IN MARCH 2007, GLORIA CRAWFORD, FIFTY, knew something was wrong. She felt a lump in her right breast, noticed associated nipple retraction and told her doctor about it. A mammogram showed an area four centimeters by three centimeters in size and an ultrasound confirmed the presence of a very large mass occupying the lateral half of the breast. Her doctor said it was a muscle mass. Gloria, a special education teacher for Chicago Public Schools, worked out nearly every day at the gym.

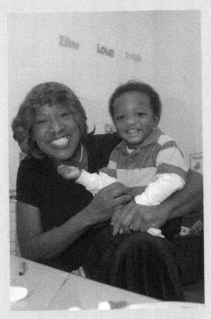

"Listen to your body. You know more than anyone whether something is wrong. Pay attention. And get a second opinion!"
—Gloria Crawford, with her grandson

Gloria finally pressed her doctor to do a biopsy, which confirmed an invasive lobular carcinoma that was ER/PR positive and HER2neu negative. Her doctor's first advice was to cut the tumor out. The thought of surgery terrified her.

"Most black women are scared to go to the doctor," Gloria said. "And when they hear cancer, they flip out. Probably all women flip out when they hear cancer...."

In April 2007, a bone scan revealed multiple areas of metastatic involvement throughout the spine, skull, and ribs. She was diagnosed as having Stage IV disease.

Gloria was started on hormone treatment with tamoxifen and began taking a drug called zoledronic acid, designed to protect her bones from the cancer.

In June 2008, Gloria came to CTCA, and was found to have a very large, seven- by eight-centimeter mass in the right breast. Since she was feeling well and responding to treatment, we simply continued the same program.

The large mass in Gloria's right breast slowly resolved. She later was changed to a different combination of hormone treatments but has not required surgery, radiation, or chemotherapy.

Nearly five years later, Gloria remains in an excellent remission on hormone therapy. There is now only a subtle area of tenderness in the right breast at the site of the original tumor, and she is virtually pain free.

While at CTCA, Gloria uses all of the available supportive services: naturopathic medicine, nutrition, acupuncture, and massage therapy. She says she's ballooned from a size ten to a size sixteen. "But who cares? I'm happy to be alive!"

Doctor's Comments

Gloria illustrates an important point that we frequently see but can't explain: that many African-American women tend to have more advanced breast cancer at the time they are first diagnosed when compared with white women.

Gloria presented with advanced (Stage IV) disease with a very large mass in the right breast and extensive spread to her bones. Lobular cancer of the breast can produce only very subtle changes on both physical examination and mammogram, and in fact Gloria had a normal mammogram in 2006—one year before she was diagnosed.

Despite the extensive amount of disease at the time of diagnosis in 2007, Gloria remains in very good health more than six years later, without aggressive treatment (no surgery, radiation, or chemotherapy).

Her story is very typical for many women with metastatic lobular carcinoma, where long remissions of excellent quality can often be achieved with relatively simple hormone therapy.

Breast Cancer in Young Women

Approximately 7 percent of women diagnosed with breast cancer are younger than forty years old at the time of diagnosis. Breast cancer in younger women poses unique diagnostic and treatment problems, both of which contribute to a poorer five-year survival rate when compared to women aged forty to fifty.

In terms of diagnosis, when a doctor sees a younger woman with a breast lump, the doctor is less likely to consider cancer as a cause of the patient's symptoms. Additionally, in younger women, normal breast tissue appears denser on a mammogram, leading to a higher rate of false-negative mammogram results for young women with a palpable breast lump. For these reasons, diagnosis is often delayed in younger women.

Diagnostic delay is particularly serious, as breast cancer in young women is often fast growing. Similar to women in the African American population, the tumors we see in the younger age group are more likely to be high grade and triple negative. Because such tumors often grow quickly, the younger patient needs prompt diagnosis, and often more aggressive treatment.

There is an additional important issue to be considered when discussing young women with breast cancer, and that is the effect of breast cancer treatment on fertility. It is unfortunately true that to effectively treat a young woman for breast cancer, we sometimes have to advise her that her plans to become pregnant have to be delayed or even abandoned altogether.

No doctor wants to deny a patient the opportunity to become a mother, but I have seen patients who refuse to take tamoxifen or end chemotherapy prematurely so that they can become pregnant. I've also seen patients halt hormone treatment because it caused a serious loss of their libido. **Refusing treatment inevitably results in an increased risk of unsuccessful treatment and a higher risk that the cancer will recur.** It is critically important that patients complete their treatment plans.

Breast cancer is a tough disease to fight in very young women. An aggressive, long-term treatment plan is often needed to provide the best chance of cure. Sometimes to ensure the very best treatment, younger patients may have to sacrifice some of their life goals. Therefore, continued emotional support of these patients is critical. This is where the support of a loving partner, and the members of our Breast Cancer Care Team can be crucial in providing appropriate emotional support.

The Contralateral (opposite) Breast

Most patients with newly diagnosed breast cancer can be cured without the need for total mastectomy, meaning complete removal of the affected breast. Regardless, some women elect to have a mastectomy rather than breast-conserving surgery. These women often ask the question, "What about my other (contralateral) breast?"

It is certainly true that women who have experienced cancer in one breast do have an increased risk for developing a new second cancer in the opposite breast in the future. And for some women, that increased risk is a source of considerable anxiety.

Cancer in the second breast is not a recurrence of the original disease, but a development of a new, second cancer entirely unrelated to the original tumor. Doctors call such a development a metachronous, contralateral breast cancer (MCBC).

It is important not to overstate the risk of developing MCBC. Reports in medical literature suggest that the lifetime risk of a new cancer developing in the opposite breast ranges from 2 percent to 11 percent. Those at higher risk are women who were younger at the time of the first cancer, have a positive family history, or had multiple tumors within the first breast. Many studies have shown that women newly diagnosed with breast cancer often greatly overestimate their risk of a future second cancer in the opposite breast.

Adjuvant hormone treatment and chemotherapy given to prevent recurrence of the original cancer also reduce the probability of MCBC. The use of a hormone treatment, such as tamoxifen, reduces that risk by 50 percent.

Here is a real example: A fifty-year-old woman with no family history of breast cancer is recently diagnosed with a three-centimeter, ER-negative/HER2neu-positive tumor with negative nodes. She elects to have a mastectomy and will then receive chemotherapy and a year of trastuzumab. She has a life expectancy of approximately thirty years and an approximate lifetime risk of developing MCBC of (at worst) approximately 10 percent.

So, if one hundred women just like her elected to remove the opposite breast to *prevent* the future development of breast cancer (we call that a *prophylactic* mastectomy), we would be removing the breasts of ninety women who would never in fact develop breast cancer.

Patient anxiety is of real concern, to be sure. I believe that when most women are presented with the numbers and realize what their true risk of MCBC is, they can be sufficiently reassured so that they decide not to proceed with removal of the second breast.

Regardless of the lower risk, some women choose to remove the opposite breast and benefit from less anxiety because of it. But there are also negative psychological effects to be considered, such as feeling self conscious, being less sexually attractive, or being dissatisfied with scars or the results of breast reconstruction.

Thirty years ago, it was almost standard practice to remove the second breast in women with lobular cancer of the breast because of an increase risk of MCBC. Thankfully, that is no longer the case. In my opinion, the only cases when serious consideration should be given to prophylactic mastectomy concern the BRCA-positive patient, or possibly the patient who underwent prior radiation for Hodgkin Disease. In these patients, the risk of a future second cancer is high enough to justify consideration of prophylactic surgery.

In cases when a patient chooses not to remove the opposite breast, she must have a clear understanding of the need for careful medical monitoring of the remaining breast.

Breast Cancer in Pregnancy and the Nursing Mother (the Lactating Breast)

Both breast cancer and pregnancy can occur in young women, so it is not surprising that some pregnant woman are newly diagnosed with breast cancer. In fact, approximately 10 percent of woman under the age of forty who are newly diagnosed with breast cancer will be pregnant at the time of diagnosis.

Although breast cancer doesn't occur very often during pregnancy (approximately one in three thousand pregnancies), it is the most common cancer occurring during pregnancy. It is very important to consider cancer in any pregnant woman who complains of a (generally painless) lump or thickening in the breast. And, it is crucial that obstetricians and gynecologists don't just *assume* that the complaint of a lump in the breast is somehow due to pregnancy.

I vividly remember a young woman with advanced breast cancer whom I saw thirty years ago. She told me that throughout her pregnancy when she complained of a lump in her breast, her obstetrician repeatedly reassured her it was simply due to her pregnancy. The day after delivery, she unbuttoned her nightgown and showed a large, ulcerated breast tumor to the doctor. By then, it was too late to save her life. To make matters worse, she was a medical student!

Because of the risk of radiation to the developing fetus, pregnant women do not have mammograms. Instead, we follow this process of diagnosis. If a pregnant woman complains of a lump in her breast, her doctor must first *think* of the possibility of breast cancer, examine her, and then order an ultrasound. If the ultrasound shows anything other than a simple cyst, it should be immediately biopsied.

Years ago, doctors thought that because of hormonal stimulation during pregnancy or some other factor, breast cancer in a pregnant woman had a worse prognosis than the same stage disease in a nonpregnant woman. Doctors also thought it best to immediately abort the fetus so that the patient could receive effective treatment for the cancer. Additionally, breast cancer in the lactating breast was also thought to carry a worse prognosis.

The truth is, in all of these cases, early diagnosis of cancer is much more difficult, and the disease is often at a more advanced stage by the time it is recognized.

When we compare cure rates for pregnant and nonpregnant women *with the same stage of disease,* the results are in fact very similar. The major contributor to the success of treating pregnant women with breast cancer is the timeliness of the diagnosis. Doctors have to *think of* breast cancer as a cause of the patient's complaints. If diagnosis and treatment are delayed due to the false assumption that it must be a cyst or an enlarged milk duct, that's when the patient gets into serious trouble.

Terminating pregnancy in order to begin effective treatment is also an obsolete recommendation. Both surgery and chemotherapy can be safely performed during pregnancy, with very little risk to mother and baby.

Treatment of the pregnant woman requires close cooperation between the surgeon, medical oncologist, and obstetrician, but a successful result with a cancer-free mother and healthy baby can certainly be achieved.

On my desk is a picture of a family—a mother, father, and several children, including the cutest little girl who was just an image on the ultrasound, while her mother was receiving chemotherapy!

Breast Cancer After Hodgkin Disease

It's one of the ironies of cancer treatment that some of the treatments we use to *cure* patients of cancer can actually *cause* cancer. The most common treatment that can actually cause cancer is probably radiation.

More than fifty years ago, radiation was used to treat young people with a variety of noncancerous conditions like enlarged tonsils, asthma, skin rashes, and even head lice. It became apparent that such treatment resulted in an increased risk of developing many cancers later in life, including cancers of the thyroid, salivary glands, and breasts. The practice of using radiation to treat noncancerous conditions has long been abandoned. However, radiation is still used to treat children and young adults with cancer.

Hodgkin Disease is a form of lymph node cancer seen in children and young adults. It frequently involves the lymph nodes in the neck and armpits and is highly curable with relatively low doses of radiation treatment. So there are many thousands of young women living today who were cured of Hodgkin Disease but exposed to radiation as part of their treatment. Unfortunately, these young women have a significantly increased risk for developing breast cancer.

There are several important points to be emphasized regarding the association of Hodgkin Disease and breast cancer:

1. Increased breast cancer risk in these patients is due to prior radiation therapy.
2. Highest risk for subsequent breast cancer is seen in those women who were treated for Hodgkin Disease when they were between ten and twenty years old (when the adolescent breast was developing).
3. The average time from radiation treatment of Hodgkin Disease until the development of breast cancer is fifteen years.
4. Most patients with breast cancer with prior Hodgkin Disease will, in all likelihood, need mastectomy. In practical terms, because of the risk of future breast cancer in the opposite breast, she may well be a candidate for bilateral mastectomy.
5. Breast cancer in patients with a past history of Hodgkin Disease is no more aggressive or less likely to be cured than breast cancer in any other patient.

Invasive Lobular Carcinoma

About 5 percent to 10 percent of all breast cancers are not the typical invasive ductal cancer, but are instead invasive lobular cancer, which can be very difficult to diagnose.

You may recall the story of Cynthia Olmstead in the introduction, a patient whose diagnosis of invasive lobular carcinoma was delayed for two years, despite the fact that she was very diligent in having regular mammograms and complained several times that she felt an abnormality in her right breast.

In contrast to invasive ductal cancer, lobular cancer often doesn't produce a discrete mass or lump in the breast. Instead, there may be only a vague area of thickening of the breast. It's not only the physical examination where abnormalities are often very subtle; the same is true for the mammogram. In fact, mammograms are frequently reported as normal in patients with lobular carcinoma, especially when the tumor is small; we rarely see calcifications in lobular carcinoma, unlike ductal cancers.

The combination of only minor abnormalities on doctors' examination and "normal" mammograms is why the diagnosis of lobular carcinoma is frequently delayed. Every woman should be suspicious if an area of her breast feels different, even if the doctor is not suspicious.

Invasive lobular cancer also has the unusual aspect of spreading to the abdomen. It's not at all unusual to see a middle-aged woman who has no complaints regarding her breasts, but complains of abdominal pain, to be diagnosed with invasive lobular cancer. When the doctors do a CAT scan, they find evidence of cancer in the liver or abdominal lymph nodes, and evidence shows metastatic lobular cancer in the biopsy of the breast.

The *treatment* of invasive lobular cancer is no different from the treatment of invasive ductal cancer, except that lobular cancer may be in multiple areas of the breast. The *prognosis* of lobular cancer is also no different from that of ductal cancer of the same stage.

Lobular Carcinoma In Situ (LCIS)

Ductal Carcinoma in Situ (DCIS) is preinvasive cancer that arises in the ducts of the breast. Treatment of DCIS is designed to prevent future development of invasive ductal carcinoma and consists of the surgical removal of the abnormal area, usually followed by radiation.

You may think a similar-sounding condition, *Lobular Carcinoma in Situ* (LCIS), is preinvasive cancer, developing in the lobule rather than in the duct, but that's not the case. LCIS is *not* preinvasive cancer; it is simply an appearance of increased growth activity in the breast that indicates an increased risk for developing breast cancer in the future. The risk of invasive cancer affects both breasts, and the future invasive cancer may be either ductal or lobular.

The lifetime risk of developing invasive cancer in the patient with LCIS should not be exaggerated. In 1990, a large study found that 16 percent (one in six) of patients with documented LCIS who received no specific treatment eventually developed invasive breast cancer.

Unlike DCIS—which may produce a lump, and often has a characteristic appearance of clusters of microscopic calcification on the mammogram—LCIS usually does not produce any symptoms or changes on the mammogram. The diagnosis is only made after a biopsy has been done to investigate some other abnormality in the breast.

After a biopsy, your doctor may not tell you that you have LCIS but may say that the biopsy showed atypical lobular hyperplasia (ALH). This is also a marker of increased proliferation very similar to LCIS, with similar significance. There is no clear agreement among doctors currently regarding how to treat patients with LCIS. Historically, options for the patient with LCIS include simple observation, bilateral prophylactic (preventive) mastectomy, or risk reduction with an estrogen-blocking drug.

Mastectomy would be considered excessive for most women with LCIS today; we generally recommend drug treatment to reduce breast cancer risk. Studies of large numbers of women conducted in the United States demonstrated a 56 percent reduction in the risk of breast cancer development in women with LCIS who were treated with tamoxifen. The study showed a similar, but slighter lower, rate of effectiveness in patients who were treated with raloxifene.

Breast Cancer in Men

Approximately 2,000 men develop breast cancer every year in the United States (approximately one man for every hundred women with the disease). The risk factors for developing male breast cancer are similar to those in women, with the addition of some uncommon diseases, where levels of testosterone are low.

In many respects, male breast cancer is like breast cancer in postmenopausal women: it occurs most commonly in men in their early sixties and is usually hormone responsive. The disease is so uncommon in men that mammographic screening of asymptomatic men is not recommended. Just like in women, the first symptom is usually a breast lump.

Because the disease is uncommon, doctors don't immediately think of cancer when a man complains of a breast lump. Thus, diagnosis is commonly delayed. The average male breast cancer measures about three centimeters (more than one inch) in diameter at the time of diagnosis. Because the male breast is much smaller than the female breast, we often see local spread of the disease into the chest wall.

The principles of treatment for men with breast cancer are the same. Any man who complains of a lump in the breast needs urgent biopsy.

Major Risk Factors for Developing Breast Cancer in Men

Genetic:
- History of breast cancer in female relative
- Ashkenazi Jewish descent
- BRCA gene mutation

Environmental exposures:
- Radiation to the breast
- Estrogen therapy

Reduced testicular function:
- Undescended testis
- Rare genetic or endocrine (glandular) diseases in which testosterone production is very low

Lifestyle factors:
- Obesity

Paget's Disease

It has been known for more than a hundred years that women (and some men) can develop a condition in which there is redness and a scaly appearance in the skin of the nipple and areola (the area immediately surrounding the nipple).

Although this condition looks just like simple inflammation of the skin (dermatitis or eczema), a biopsy of the affected skin shows abnormal cells that represent carcinoma in situ (noninvasive cancer).

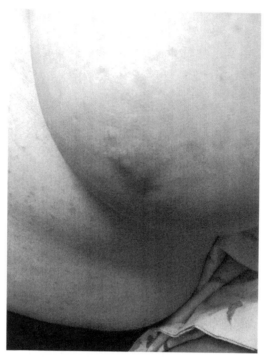

Paget's Disease of the nipple. This patient complained of pain, itching, and burning.

The importance of recognizing that the changes of Paget's Disease are not simply dermatitis is the fact that a cancer is found in the underlying breast of more than 97 percent of patients with Paget's Disease of the nipple.

Only about half of the patients with Paget's Disease have a mass in the breast, and most of those who don't have a mass will have an entirely normal mammogram. MRI of the breast may be useful in identifying areas of cancer in the breast that can't be felt or seen on mammogram.

The lesson: If you ever develop changes in the skin of the nipple, you must immediately see your doctor. Doctors who see a patient with such skin changes must have a high degree of suspicion and refer the patient for a biopsy of the affected nipple.

Treatment of Paget's Disease is surgical removal of the affected area and of the underlying cancer, and it is generally very successful.

Brain Metastasis

One of the greatest difficulties for patients with breast cancer occurs when the disease spreads into the brain or the tissues that surround the brain (the meninges).

Brain metastases are more common in patients with HER2-positive or triple-negative breast cancer (high-grade tumors). They are also more likely to develop in women with inflammatory breast cancer, African-American women, younger women, and those who have achieved a long remission from metastatic disease elsewhere in the body.

There are several reasons why patients with advanced breast cancer may develop brain or meningeal metastases.

The brain is such a critically important organ that it is protected from many potentially harmful chemicals that may find their way into our blood by (the blood-brain barrier). Many drugs can cross the blood-brain barrier, including general anesthetics, morphine, and alcohol. However, most chemotherapy drugs don't enter into the brain. As a result, cancer cells can find a sanctuary within the brain in patients with advanced breast cancer.

It is ironic that, as our treatment of patients with Stage IV breast cancer has become more effective and such patients are living longer, we are seeing more of them develop brain metastases.

There is no question that the development of brain metastases has a negative effect on the chances of long-term survival. Drug treatment is generally not effective, so some form of radiation is generally recommended.

There are some hopeful developments, however. We know that women with HER2- positive breast cancer metastatic to the brain are much more likely to respond well to treatment. Lapatinib, a drug that crosses the blood-brain barrier, has been very active against

HER2-positive breast cancer and offers the possibility of long-term control of disease.

Additionally specific genetic alterations have recently been identified that may allow us to identify women who have breast cancers that are particularly likely to develop brain metastases.

Currently, we use prophylactic (preventive) radiation to the brain in patients with lung cancers that are associated with a high rate of relapse. It is possible that a similar approach may be used in some patients with breast cancer in the future to prevent what remains a very difficult clinical problem.

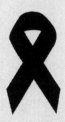

Still Going Strong, Five Years after Brain Metastases

IN JANUARY 2005, WHEN DONNA CISTARO WAS ONLY THIRTY-EIGHT YEARS OLD, she discovered a lump in her left breast. With no family history, she was baffled. "It felt like someone was pulling the muscle away from the breast bone," Donna explains.

Born and raised in Indiana, Donna went to see her family doctor, who sent her for a mammogram and then to meet with a surgeon. She chose to be treated in Chicago, at a hospital where her cousin worked. There, she underwent a left mastectomy, followed by chemotherapy and treatment using tamoxifen.

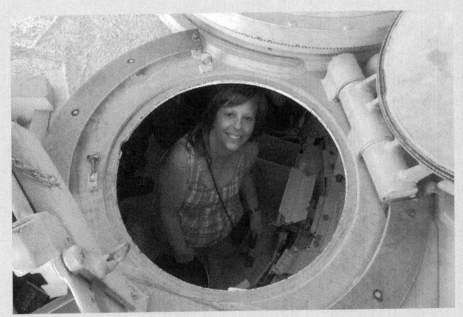

"This cancer is not going to get me. I'm too young. I'm not ready to leave."
— *Donna Cistaro*

Two years later, Donna developed a dry cough and chest pain. "I went to my family doctor. They thought I had walking pneumonia and gave me antibiotics, but I just wasn't getting better. He finally did an X-ray and said, 'This is not pneumonia.'"

Donna returned to Chicago. "Even though my cousin was there, I didn't like the hospital," she says. "Everything was dirty. Two ladies my age who also had cancer had passed away. When the radiation doctor said, 'You know, the type of cancer you have is going to kill you,' I had to get out of there," she says. "All I could think of was, 'Who is going to raise my kids?'"

In June 2007, Donna came to CTCA at Midwestern and became my patient. CAT scans at that time showed that her cancer had spread to her lungs, liver, and bone. "No one had ever told me that I had eight tumors in my liver."

Donna was treated with chemotherapy. Since her cancer was positive for HER2neu, she also received trastuzumab, followed by an experimental drug targeting HER2neu. Because of this treatment, her lung and liver metastases quickly resolved.

One year later, she was found to have two brain metastases, which required pinpoint radiation. Today, Donna comes to the hospital once per month and receives a combination of trastuzumab and a new HER2 targeted therapy called pertuzumab to keep the cancer in remission.

In June 2012, Donna celebrated with other five-year cancer survivors. She touches her name plaque on the Celebrate Life tree every time she visits. At the time I'm writing this in September 2013, Donna is still very active, nearly nine years after her initial diagnosis.

"I never in a million years thought I'd see my name on that tree," she says proudly.

Doctor's Comments

Approximately 20 percent of breast cancers contain the growth factor HER2neu. Such tumors are biologically aggressive and more likely to recur than HER2-negative breast cancer. They are also more likely to spread to the brain.

The good news about HER2-positive disease is that there are now at least five very active drugs available that specifically target the HER2 protein, or the cellular processes related to it. Because these drugs are very specific in their action, they are very effective and less likely to cause severe side effects than older chemotherapy drugs.

In previous years, patients whose breast cancers spread to the brain had very limited survival rates, but those poor prognoses have been greatly improved with newer radiation techniques and drug treatments, as Donna's experience illustrates.

Bone Metastases

When cancer cells metastasize and spread from the breast into distant areas of the body through the blood stream (described in Chapter 2), they frequently settle in the skeleton. Bone marrow apparently provides an environment very favorable for the growth of cancer cells.

If undetected and untreated, these cells grow and eventually produce secondary tumors, metastases in the bone itself. Bone metastases are seen most frequently in the axial skeleton (pelvis, spine, ribs, and skull bone), rather than the peripheral skeleton (forearm, lower leg, small bones of the hand and feet).

There are two basic types of bone metastases: *osteolytic* and *osteoblastic* metastases. The difference can be seen in X-ray studies. In osteolytic metastases, the cancer cells destroy the bone, producing holes in the bone. In osteoblastic metastases, there is little bone destruction, but the bone responds to the presence of cancer cells by forming new bone, creating a denser than normal appearance on X-ray.

These two different effects have important clinical distinctions. All bone metastases can cause bone pain, but because of the extent of bone destruction, osteolytic metastases are more likely to cause fractures of affected bone (usually in weight-bearing bones like the spine or thigh bone). We call a fracture in a bone weakened by cancer a *pathologic fracture*. Such fractures can occur with little or no history of injury.

Osteolytic metastases are also more likely to cause hypercalcemia, a rise in blood calcium levels that can cause serious problems like vomiting, dehydration, and kidney damage.

Sometimes patients with bone metastases will need specific palliative treatment to relieve severe pain, or even a surgical procedure by an orthopedic or spine surgeon to prevent or treat a fracture. Radiation is often very effective in relieving pain caused by bone metastases.

The best treatment for bone metastases is to control the underlying disease using drug treatment. As many patients with bone metastases have ER-positive breast cancer, hormone therapy is often very effective.

In recent years, several new drugs have become available that are able to effectively prevent breast cancer cells in bone from destroying the bone. Although drugs like pamidronic acid, zoledronic acid, and denosumab do not directly kill the cancer cells, they will prevent bone damage and hypercalcemia, particularly when combined with effective chemotherapy or hormone therapy.

A Message of Hope

"Breast cancer meant I had to rely on others, learn to let go of everything, realize what was truly meaningful and important to the deepest core of my being, and learn to trust my doctors. I would have not chosen to have breast cancer, but I am thankful for the experiences I have had that have helped shape me into the woman I am now."
— *Teri Wentworth*

I want to finish this book with a message of hope for all women.

There have been tremendous advances in our understanding and treatment of breast cancer over the past fifty years. Consider these facts:

In the decade 1944 to 1954, only 16 percent of women with breast cancer that had spread to the lymph nodes were alive ten years after diagnosis. In the decade 1995 to 2004, that percentage had risen to 74 percent, representing a five-fold increase. Our treatments today are even more effective. And as treatments have become more effective, they have also become much more tolerable, with far fewer long-term side effects for the patient.

There is a huge disconnect in this country, however. When I attend medical meetings regarding breast cancer, I hear doctors discuss the results of high-powered scientific research in molecular biology, breast cancer genetics, improved imaging technology, and the most advanced treatments for breast cancer. There is no doubt that we have made tremendous advances in our knowledge and treatment of this disease. Yet too many women are still denying themselves the benefits of these advances by delaying diagnosis or refusing to use established and proven treatments.

That is the reason I wrote this book. I want women and the families who love them to understand that breast cancer is a very curable disease, and I believe our greatest weapon against breast cancer is education. The more every woman understands the disease, and how doctors and modern medicine work to fight it, the better we will be able to treat it, to cure it, and to keep it in remission.

My heartfelt advice to all women facing breast cancer is this: If you want to explore alternative treatments to complement traditional treatment, that's fine. I sincerely believe that an integrative approach combining the latest conventional treatment with the best of natural, holistic measures in a supportive role will provide you with the best chance for cure of your breast cancer, while maintaining optimal physical and mental health. But please don't refuse surgery, radiation, and drug treatments that offer you a cure of this disease.

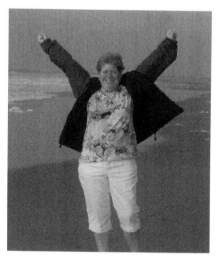

Breast cancer survivor Diane Butler-Hughes

I hope health professionals read this book too because we in the health care profession also need education. Primary care doctors on the front lines of early diagnosis need to understand the limitations of clinical examination and current imaging techniques like mammograms.

And doctors and other health professionals who treat women with breast cancer need additional education. We must recognize that we have a tremendous responsibility to each patient, to listen to her concerns and be respectful of her beliefs. Her beliefs may not be our beliefs, and they may be incompatible with our understanding of the medical science. But we cannot simply dismiss them. When we dismiss a patient's beliefs, we run the risk of having the patient refuse conventional treatment and look elsewhere for a solution.

We must always remember that our patients are very frightened. We need to remain kind and compassionate at all times. We need to do our best to communicate effectively with our colleagues, our patients, and their families.

Patients cannot cure themselves of cancer. Every woman with breast cancer has to find a team of doctors that she trusts and follow their advice. It is our job as a health care team to earn that trust every day.

Every health care professional who treats a woman with breast cancer has a responsibility to educate her and to guide her to make the best treatment choices that are consistent with her personal values and her medical condition. For this is the only way that she, as the patient, can receive the highest assurance of the best possible outcome.

Acknowledgments

Treatment of the patient with breast cancer is very much a team effort, and I'm fortunate to be part of a great team. I would like to thank all of the health care professionals in the Breast Cancer Treatment Team at Cancer Treatment Centers of America® (CTCA®) at Midwest Regional Medical Center (Midwestern). Their dedication to each and every patient is truly remarkable.

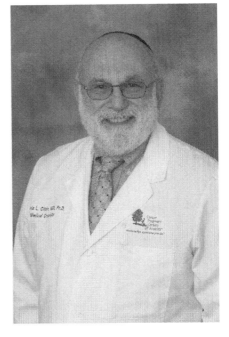

I would like to thank the Administration at Midwestern for their encouragement and support, in particular Anne Meisner (now leading CTCA at Southeastern Regional Medical Center), Scott Jones, and Pete Govorchin.

I'm grateful to Maurie Markman, MD, Senior Vice President of Clinical Affairs at CTCA; Edgar Staren, MD, PhD, President and CEO of CTCA at Western Regional Medical Center, breast surgeon, and past President of the American Society of Breast Surgeons; Bradford Tan, MD, National Director of Pathology and Laboratory Medicine; Carolyn Lammersfeld, MS, RD, CSO, LD, CNSC, Vice President of Integrative Medicine at CTCA; and Christina Shannon, ND, FABNO, Clinical

Director of Naturopathic Medicine for their contributions, insight, and important constructive criticism of the manuscript.

I would like to thank my patient and fine artist Terrece Crawford for providing the illustrations for this book.

Our research efforts at Midwestern provided some of the data presented in this book, and it's a pleasure to acknowledge the hard work and input of James Grutsch, PhD, and Sara Mortensen, BA, in our research projects.

Writing this book has taken up much of my free time, and I would like to thank my dear wife, Rena, for her patience and encouragement.

Special thanks to my outstanding editor, Catherine Driscoll, who has magically turned this sow's ear into what I hope is a silk purse (or approximation thereof!). A special thanks to Mary Alice Horstman, Director of Public Affairs at Midwestern, for her tireless efforts to keep the project running smoothly, and to Cathy Santos and Jackie Carey for their continued support.

Finally, the focus at CTCA is always on the patient. I want to thank all of my patients for their contributions. Many patients shared their journeys and graciously permitted me to tell their stories. I hope that these stories have educated and inspired you, as much as they inspire me every day. I dedicate this book to all of my patients.

Important Questions to Ask Your Doctors

The modern approach to breast cancer diagnosis and treatment requires that all of the relevant information regarding cancer stage and type be gathered before treatment is started. To make the most educated decisions, a patient should meet with her surgeon, medical oncologist, and radiation therapist to discuss the information gathered and plan the best course of treatment.

In many cases, it's entirely possible to avoid mastectomy altogether. But if a woman must have a mastectomy, she should meet with a plastic (reconstructive) surgeon to discuss her options for breast reconstruction before the primary surgery. Remember, a mastectomy is an irreversible procedure, even with breast reconstruction. It's critically important that every woman be fully informed of all options before starting treatment.

Last, every woman has to be her own advocate. You are not being pushy or obnoxious by asking questions. You're being responsible. It is your right to know every detail that is relevant to your care. Below are some questions to guide you in your conversations with doctors.

Ask all doctors the following questions:

- What stage is my cancer?
- What type of breast cancer do I have?
- Have you spoken to the other doctors in my team about your recommendations?
- Are you all in agreement with the treatment plan?

You should ask the cancer surgeon these specific questions:

- What surgical options do I have?
- What surgical option do you recommend?
- Why do you recommend that?
- Would drug treatment before surgery help to shrink the tumor?
- If not, why not?
- Do you offer intraoperative radiation as an option?
- Do you have a postoperative rehab program available? May I meet them before surgery?

If your surgeon recommends removing the entire breast, you should also ask about the following:

- I understand that most women don't need to have the entire breast removed, and that the cure rate is no higher for mastectomy compared with lumpectomy. So why do you recommend removing the entire breast?

If your surgeon recommends removing both breasts, you should ask the following questions:

- If there is no cancer in my other breast, what is my lifetime risk of developing a cancer in the other breast?
- What is the scientific basis for that number?
  Here are some questions to ask your plastic (reconstructive) surgeon:
- What are my options for surgical reconstruction?
- Which option do you recommend?
- Why do you recommend that?
- I understand that radiation may be needed after surgery. What would that mean for reconstruction?

Below are specific questions to ask the medical oncologist:

Based on the stage and type of breast cancer that I have, what drug treatment are you recommending?

- Why do you recommend this?
- What are the alternatives?
- Would drug treatment before surgery be helpful to shrink the tumor?
- If not, why not?
- Do you agree with surgeon's recommendations?
- I understand that after surgery you may have more information about my cancer. If your treatment recommendations change will we have adequate time to discuss them?

If your surgeon recommends removing the entire breast, you should also ask the following question:

- I understand that most women don't need to have the entire breast removed, and that the cure rate is no higher for mastectomy compared with lumpectomy. So why is my surgeon recommending removing the entire breast?

Ask your radiation oncologist the following specific questions:

- Will I need radiation as part of my treatment?
- What radiation options are available for me?
- Is intraoperative radiation an option for me?
- What radiation do you recommend for my case and why?
- Have you spoken with my surgeons (including reconstructive surgeon)?

Glossary of Terms

Adjuvant Therapy refers to drug treatment given for a limited time after surgical removal of a breast tumor. Adjuvant therapy is given to patients who have no evidence of residual cancer, but are considered to be at high risk for developing recurrent cancer because of the presence of one or more negative prognostic factors. Adjuvant drug treatment is given to kill any occult metastatic disease that may be present.

Biologic typing determines what type of cancer is present and has an important influence on prognosis and treatment. There a number of different factors that doctors measure in a breast cancer sample to help determine the biologic type of breast cancer.

Biopsy is a procedure where a sample of the breast tissue from any area in question is removed and examined under a microscope. Biopsy will confirm whether a suspicious lump is indeed cancerous and also can provide a great deal of information regarding the biologic type of the cancer.

BRCA 1 and 2 are the most important gene mutations that doctors test for when they suspect that a patient may have familial breast cancer. These gene mutations should be suspected when breast cancer occurs in patients with strong family history of breast and/or ovarian cancer, under age forty, in men, in Jewish patients, and in patients with triple-negative breast cancer.

Carcinomas are cancers that form in the lining tissue of organs. Most common cancers, include breast cancer, are carcinomas.

Comorbidities are other medical conditions unrelated to the cancer that may affect the patient's ability to receive effective breast cancer treatment. Examples of significant comorbidities would be severe heart failure or diabetes.

Cure of breast cancer is defined as total removal and destruction of all evident breast cancer with absence of tumor recurrence during the remainder of the patient's lifetime. Most women diagnosed today with early stage breast cancer can confidently expect to be cured of their disease if they receive appropriate treatment and follow that treatment completely.

Cytotoxic Chemotherapy refers to chemicals (drugs) that are cytotoxic, meaning they damage and can kill living cells. There are a large number of chemotherapy drugs that can kill breast cancer cells, and doctors have used such drugs for more than fifty years in the treatment of patients with breast cancer.

Diagnostic mammogram is an X-ray examination that focuses on a specific area in one breast, and is often done with magnification of the particular area of interest. Diagnostic mammogram may follow a screening mammogram.

Ductal Carcinoma in Situ (DCIS) is preinvasive breast cancer in which cancer cells form inside the milk ducts in the breast but have not yet invaded outside the over into surrounding the breast issue. DCIS is often recognized on the mammogram by the presence of microscopic areas of calcification and can often be identified through a screening mammogram long before true, invasive breast cancer is present.

Estrogen is a sex hormone, a chemical produced in the ovary that stimulates normal breast cells and some breast cancer cells to grow.

Estrogen and Progesterone Receptors (ER/PR) are estrogen-binding proteins present in estrogen sensitive cells in the normal breast. Estrogen binds to the cell through the estrogen receptor, stimulating the breast cell to divide. Some breast cancer cells also contain high levels of ER. ER-positive breast cancers are biologically less aggressive than ER-negative breast cancers and are often effectively treated with endocrine treatment. Progesterone Receptor, or PR, is less important biologically and clinically than estrogen receptor.

Familial Breast Cancer Approximately 10 percent of all breast cancers occur in women who have close relatives (mother, grandmother, sister) with a history of breast cancer. A history of breast or ovarian cancer in a family member should raise the possibility of familial breast cancer. Many different genes increase breast cancer risk. The two most common are mutations of BRCA1 and BRCA2.

Genes are an essential component of all living cells. Genes direct cells to function in specific ways. They contain DNA and RNA and are sometimes referred to as the building blocks of life. Cancer cells contain abnormal genes.

Genomic Testing describes a process in which breast cancer tissue is tested in the laboratory to determine the specific genes, which it contains. Genomic testing provides doctors with important information regarding the future behavior of a cancer and also may identify treatment that will target a specific target gene in the cancer.

Gynecomastia is swelling and tenderness of the breasts in men and is seen as a side effect of some treatments for prostate cancer.

Hormone or Endocrine Treatment of breast cancer refers to treatment of patients with estrogen receptor positive breast cancer. Endocrine treatments are designed to reduce to a minimum the stimulation of growth of breast cancer cells by the female sex hormone estrogen.

Invasive Breast Carcinoma develops when breast cancer cells penetrate the walls of the milk ducts and invade the surrounding fatty tissue of the breast.

Inflammatory Breast Cancer is a special type of breast cancer that produces redness of the skin of the breast. It should be considered in any woman who has what appears to be a breast infection, particularly if the "infection" doesn't clear up rapidly with antibiotics.

Lobular Carcinoma is a special type of breast cancer that may be difficult to diagnose for two reasons. First, lobular carcinoma often doesn't produce an obvious lump in the breast; it often just causes a subtle area of thickening in the breast that many doctors find unimpressive when they examine the patient. Second, lobular cancer often doesn't show up on the mammogram.

Locoregional recurrence refers to breast cancer that recurs, sometimes years after initial treatment, in the breast, axilla (armpit), or chest wall near where the original cancer was located.

Lymph Nodes are located throughout the body. They form part of the immune system and play a role in fighting infections. Lymph nodes are also an important location where cancer cells spread. The lymph nodes in the armpit (axilla) are often the first place breast cancer cells spread to when they leave the breast. Testing the axillary nodes for cancer cells is an important part of the staging of early breast cancer.

Lymphedema is a condition where there is swelling of the arm following surgical removal of or radiation to the lymph nodes in the axilla (armpit). Lymphedema may persist for years.

Mastectomy is the surgical operation where the entire breast is surgically removed. It is often combined with surgical removal of one or more axillary lymph nodes.

Metastases are secondary tumors formed when breast cancer cells spread through the lymphatic system or the blood stream to areas distant from the breast. Metastases from a cancer of the breast may be found in lymph nodes in the axilla (armpit), or in distant organs like lung, liver, bone, and brain.

Metachronous contralateral breast cancer refers to the development of a new cancer in the opposite breast, usually many years after successful treatment for breast cancer. Patients with BRCA gene mutations are most likely to develop a second cancer in the opposite breast.

Neoadjuvant therapy refers to drug treatment given before surgery for breast cancer. Neoadjuvant therapy will often significantly shrink the cancer, thus allowing the surgeon to remove much less breast tissue at the time of surgery. Many patients who would otherwise need mastectomy can have breast-conserving surgery when neoadjuvant drug treatment is given first.

Occult metastatic disease occurs when the cancer spreads to distant parts of the body before the primary cancer in the breast has been identified or removed. These cells are usually undetectable when breast cancer is first diagnosed, but will grow silently to cause later relapse.

Palliation refers to medical treatment given to relieve a patient's symptoms.

Prognosis refers to the probability of a future positive result (cure or long-term remission) or the opposite. It is a doctor's best estimate, based on all of the medical facts available, of what is likely to happen in the future. In patients with newly diagnosed breast cancer, prognosis is based on the stage and the biologic type of the disease.

Recurrent or relapse of breast cancer occurs months or years after initial diagnosis and treatment, when the growth of occult metastatic disease has reached a critical mass that allows the clinical identification of recurrence.

Screening mammogram is an X-ray of the breasts of women who have no breast complaints. Regular screening mammograms form an important strategy for improving a woman's probability of preventing death from breast cancer through early diagnosis.

Staging of cancer is the process through which doctors identify how much cancer is present in a patient, and exactly where it is present in the body.

Symptoms are feelings that a patient experiences that are caused by an illness. In the case of breast cancer, the most common symptom is feeling a lump in the breast. Other symptoms include pain caused by cancer spread into bones, and shortness of breath caused by cancerous fluid around the lungs.

Systemic recurrence refers to breast cancer that recurs as metastases in distant organs, such as lung, liver, or bone.

Targeted therapy refers to drug treatment that attacks a specific target gene or protein within a breast cancer cell. Targeted therapies have been very successful in treating breast cancer, and are less likely to cause side effects than cytotoxic chemotherapy. Examples of targeted therapy include tamoxifen, which targets the estrogen receptor, and trastuzumab, which attacks HER2neu.

Treatment side effects are unwanted symptoms or damage occurring as a result of treatment. Side effects can be as trivial as fatigue after chemotherapy, or (rarely) can be severe or even life threatening. Every doctor who recommends a treatment to the patient must always consider possible side effects and balance the risks of treatment against the benefits.

Triple-Negative Breast Cancer is a special type of breast cancer that is seen most frequently in very young women, in patients with BRCA mutations and in African-American women. "Triple negative" refers to the fact that these cancers do not contain estrogen or progesterone receptor (ER or PR) or the growth factor HER2neu. Triple-negative breast cancers are generally rapidly growing tumors that are highly susceptible to chemotherapy.

Tumor grade describes how the appearance of the cancer looks under the microscope and usually is described on a scale of one to three (low to high grade). Low-grade breast cancers are generally less biologically aggressive than high-grade cancers.

Ultrasound examination of an area of concern in the breast is often used if a woman complains of a lump or mass in her breast. The ultrasound frequently allows the doctor to distinguish between a solid mass and a fluid-filled structure (cyst), which is much less likely to be cancerous.

Common Drugs Used in Breast Cancer Treatment

Generic	Brand Name
Ado-trastuzumab emtansine	Kadcyla(TDM-1)
Anastrozole	Arimidex
Capecitabine	Xeloda
Carboplatin	Paraplatin
Cetuximab	Erbitux
Cisplatin	Platinol
Cyclophosphamide	Cytoxan
Denosumab	Xgeva
Docetaxel	Taxotere
Doxorubicin	Adriamycin
Doxorubicin liposomal	Doxil
Eribulin	Halaven
Everolimus	Afinitor
Exemestane	Aromasin
Gemcitabine	Gemzar
Ixabepilone	Ixempra
Lapatinib	Tykerb
Letrozole	Femera
Neratinib	
Paclitaxel	Taxol
Paclitaxel protein-bound	Abraxane
Pamidronic acid	Aredia
Pertuzumab	Perjeta
Raloxifene	Evista
Tamoxifen	Nolvadex
Trastuzumab	Herceptin
Vinorelbine	Navelbine
Zoledronic acid	Zometa

Patient Resources & Information

These organizations provide breast cancer information, counseling, publications, advocacy, support, and referral services.

American Association of Naturopathic Providers (AANP) www.naturopathic.org. The AANP is the national professional society representing licensed naturopathic physicians. AANP's physician members are graduates of naturopathic medical schools accredited by the Council on Naturopathic Medical Education. CNME is recognized by the US Department of Education as the national accrediting agency for programs leading to the Doctor of Naturopathic Medicine (ND or NMD) or Doctor of Naturopathy (ND) degree.

American Cancer Society (ACS): cancer.org or 800-227-2345. Website and twenty-four-hour hotline provide information on cancer treatment, early detection, prevention, and online services available to patients with cancer and their families.

Association of Cancer Online Resources: acor.org. The Association provides information and support to patients with cancer and those who take care of them through the creation and maintenance of cancer-related Internet mailing lists, web-based resources, an email forum and a discussion group.

American Institute for Cancer Research: aicr.org. The American Institute for Cancer Research was founded on a simple but radical idea:

that everyday choices can reduce our chances of getting cancer. AICR is a great resource that focuses on the link between diet and cancer, and translating the results into practical information for the public.

Cancer Treatment Centers of America (CTCA): cancercenter.org or 800-333-CTCA. Cancer Treatment Centers of America® (CTCA) is a national network of hospitals focusing on complex and advanced-stage cancer. CTCA® offers a comprehensive, fully integrated approach to cancer treatment and serves patients from all fifty states at hospitals located in Atlanta, Chicago, Philadelphia, Phoenix, and Tulsa. Known for delivering the Mother Standard® of care and Patient Empowerment Medicine®, CTCA provides patients with information about cancer and their treatment options, so they can control their treatment decisions.

Cancer Care Inc.: cancercare.org or 800-813-HOPE. Cancer Care provides free counseling and emotional support, information on medical care and treatment, and help with financial aspects of care; this includes referral to online, telephone, and in-person assistance.

Facing Our Risk of Cancer Empowered: facingourrisk.org or 866-288-7475. Facing Our Risk of Cancer Empowered (FORCE) is a nonprofit organization for women who are at high risk of getting breast and ovarian cancers due to their family history and genetic status, and for members of families in which a BRCA mutation may be present.

Inflammatory Breast Cancer Research Foundation: ibcresearch.org or 877-786-7422. The IBC Research Foundation specifically targets IBC and the research to find its cause.

Living Beyond Breast Cancer: lbbc.org or 888-753-5222. On this site you will find current and past issues of this organization's newsletter, transcripts of past educational programs, and information about a toll-free survivors' helpline, which is staffed by breast cancer survivors. There is also information about a young survivors' network.

Look Good...Feel Better: lookgoodfeelbetter.org or 800-395-LOOK. Look Good...Feel Better is dedicated to improving the self-esteem and quality of life of people undergoing treatment for cancer. It is their aim to improve their self-image and appearance through complimentary group, individual and self-help beauty sessions that create a sense of support, confidence, courage, and community.

National Cancer Institute (NCI): cancernet.nci.nih.gov, cancer.gov or 800-422-6237. NCI, a federal government agency which is the largest division of the National Institutes of Health, conducts and supports research, training, dissemination of health information and other programs with respect to the cause, diagnosis, prevention and treatment of cancer, rehabilitation from cancer and the continuing care of patients with cancer and their families. The websites and phone line provide information on all of these aspects. Up-to-date information on clinical trials also can be found at cancertrials.nci.nih.gov.

National Coalition for Cancer Survivorship (NCCS): canceradvocacy. org or 877-622-7937. NCCS is a national advocacy group for people with all types of cancer and those who care for them. The site has hyperlinks, legislative news, and information on clinical trials.

National Society of Genetic Counselors: nsgc@nsgc.org, 312-321-6834. The American Board of Genetic Counseling certifies genetic counselors and accredits genetic counseling training programs. For information about genetic risk of cancer, see also the American Cancer Society, and National Cancer Institute Cancer Genetics Overview (PDQ®) at http://www.cancer.gov/cancertopics/pdq/genetics/overview.

Oncology Association of Naturopathic Physicians (OncANP) www.oncanp.org. The OncANP is a professional association of naturopathic physicians with a focus on treating individuals diagnosed with cancer. The board certification body of the Oncology Association of Naturopathic Physicians is the American Board of Naturopathic Oncology (ABNO) and this board oversees the testing and certification process for naturopathic physicians in naturopathic oncology.

Reach To Recovery: cancer.org. Reach To Recovery is a program of the American Cancer Society to help people (female and male) cope with their breast cancer experience. Volunteers are breast cancer survivors who give patients and family members an opportunity to express feelings, talk about fears and concerns, and ask questions of someone who is knowledgeable and level headed.

ShareCare: sharecare.com. ShareCare is an interactive platform that provides expert health information and allows you to ask questions and get answers from trusted health care experts.

SHARE: sharecancersupport.org or 212-719-0364/866-891-2392. Self-help for women with breast or ovarian cancer. SHARE provides information hotlines in English and Spanish, peer-led support groups, public education, and advocacy and wellness programs.

Sharsheret: Sharsheret.org. Sharsheret is a national not-for-profit organization supporting young women and their families of all Jewish backgrounds facing breast cancer. The mission of Sharsheret is to offer a community of support to women diagnosed with breast cancer or ovarian cancer, at increased genetic risk, by fostering culturally relevant individualized connections with networks of peers, health professionals, and related resources.

Sisters Network, Inc.: sistersnetworkinc.org. Sisters Network is a national African-American breast cancer survivors' organization that provides support networks and cancer prevention programs.

Susan G. Komen for the Cure®: komen.org or 877-465-6636. Susan G. Komen for the Cure® was established in 1982, launching a global breast cancer movement. Events like the Komen Race for the Cure have allowed Komen to invest almost two billion dollars to fulfill its promise, working to end breast cancer in the United States and throughout the world through ground-breaking research, community health outreach, advocacy and programs in more than fifty countries. Since 1982, Komen has played a critical role in every major advance in the fight against breast cancer—transforming how the world talks about and treats this disease and helping to turn millions of patients with breast cancer into breast cancer survivors.

The Sister Study: sisterstudy.org. The Sister Study is the only long-term study of women aged thirty-five to seventy-four whose sisters had breast cancer. It is a national study to learn how environment and genes affect the chances of getting breast cancer. In the next three years, fifty thousand women whose sister had breast cancer and who do not have breast cancer themselves will be asked to join the study.

The Witness Project: 203-367-4432. This organization recruits and trains African-American breast and cervical cancer survivors to become witness role models. These witness role models provide culturally appropriate educational and empowerment messages in sessions at African-American churches and community centers to promote the practice of breast self-examination, mammography, clinical breast examination, and Pap test screening.

Triple-Negative Breast Cancer Foundation: tnbcfoundation.org. This organization's mission is to raise awareness of triple-negative breast cancer and to support scientists and researchers determine the definitive causes of triple-negative breast cancer so that effective detection, diagnosis, prevention, and treatment can be pursued.

Suggested Further Reading

Hopefully, this book has empowered you by describing the different types of breast cancer and the available treatments. Below is a list of articles and websites that provide additional information and the results of scientific studies that support many of the opinions expressed in this book.

Please note that these sources are written for medical professionals, so they are typically written in highly technical language. I don't recommend that any patient or family member try to use any of these resources to develop their own treatment plan.

There is an enormous amount of medical literature on breast cancer, with thousands of articles being published every year. This list is in no way comprehensive but is offered as a guide for the interested reader to find articles related to specific topics.

If you have specific questions, you are encouraged to seek answers from your doctors.

Breast Cancer Statistics

Siegel R, Naishadham D, Jemal A, "Cancer statistics," 2012, CA: *A Cancer Journal for Clinicians 2011,* http://dx.doi.org/10.3322/caac.20138

Breast Cancer Staging

Edge SB, Byrd, DR Compton CC, et al., eds. *AJCC Cancer Staging Manual 7th Edition* New York : Springer 2010.

"Baseline Staging Tests in Primary Breast Cancer: Practice Guideline Report # 1-14: Members of the Breast Cancer Disease Site Group" http://www.cancercare.on.ca/common/pages/UserFile. asp?serverId=6&path=/File%20Database/CCO%20Files/PEBC/ pebc1-14.pdf. Accessed

Biology of Breast Cancer

"Genomics-Based Prognosis and Therapeutic Prediction in Breast Cancer," *Journal of National Comprehensive Cancer Network* 2005, 3 291-300 590 http://www.ncbi.nlm.nih.gov/pubmed/16002001

"The Distinctive Nature of HER2-Positive Breast Cancers," Burstein HJ, *New England Journal of Medicine* 2005 353 1652-1654. 590 http://www. ncbi.nlm.nih.gov/pubmed/16236735

"Advances in Breast Cancer: Pathways to Personalized Medicine," Olopade OI, Grushko TA, Nanda R, et al., *Clinical Cancer Research* 2008, Volume 14, Page 7988

"Metastatic Potential of T1 Breast Cancer Can Be Predicted by the 70-Gene MammaPrint Signature," Mook, S., Knauer, M., Bueno-de-Mesquita JM, et al., *Annals of Surgical Oncology 2010* 17 1406-1413 590 http://www.ncbi.nlm.nih.gov/pubmed/20094918

Signs and Symptoms of Breast Cancer

Osteen, R. Breast Cancer. In: Lenhard RE, Osteen RT, Gansler R, eds. Clinical Oncology. Atlanta, GA: American Cancer Society; 2001:251–268.

Diagnostic Evaluation of a Breast Lump

"Evaluation of Palpable Breast Masses," Klein S, American Family Physician. 2005 71 (9):1731-1738.

"Diagnostic Evaluation of Women with Suspected Breast Cancer," Esserman LJ, Joe BN http://www.uptodate.com/contents/diagnostic-evaluation-of-women-with-suspected-breast-cancer

Mammograms

"Efficacy of Screening Mammography: A Meta-Analysis," Kerlikowske K, Grady D, Rubin SM, et al., *Journal of the American Medical Association* 1995 273(2)149-154. doi:10.1001/jama.1995.03520260071035.

"Swedish Two-County Trial: Impact of Mammographic Screening on Breast Cancer Mortality During Three Decades," Duffy SW, Tabar L, Vitak B, et al., *Radiology*. 2011;doi:10.1148/radiol.11110469.

Surgery

"Nipple-Sparing Mastectomy: Evaluation of Patient Satisfaction, Aesthetic Results, and Sensation," *Annals of Plastic Surgery* 2009 62 586-590, http://www.ncbi.nlm.nih.gov/pubmed/19387167

"Benefit or Bias? The Role of Surgery to Remove the Primary Tumor in Patients with Metastatic Breast Cancer," Olson JA, Marcom PK, *Annals of Surgery* 2008 247 739-740 http://www.ncbi.nlm.nih.gov/pubmed/18438109

"A Randomized Comparison of Sentinel-Bode Biopsy with Routine Axillary Dissection in Breast Cancer," Veronesi U, Paganelli G, Viale G, et al., *New England Journal of Medicine* 2003 349 546-553 http://www.ncbi.nlm.nih.gov/pubmed/12904519

Breast Reconstruction

Ahmed S, Snelling A, Bains M, Whitworth IH, *British Medical Journal* 2005 330 943-948, http://www.ncbi.nlm.nih.gov/pubmed/15845976

Radiation Treatment

"Twenty-Year Follow-Up of a Randomized Trial Comparing Total Mastectomy, Lumpectomy, and Lumpectomy Plus Irradiation for the Treatment of Invasive Breast Cancer," *New England Journal of Medicine* 2002 347 1233-1241 http://www.nejm.org/doi/full/10.1056/NEJMoa022152

"Effects of Radiotherapy and of Differences the Extent of Surgery for Early Breast Cancer on Local Recurrences and 15-year Survival: An Overview of the Randomised Trials," Clarke M, Collins R, Darby S, et al.
Lancet 2005 366 2087-2106 http://www.ncbi.nlm.nih.gov/pubmed/16360786

Medical Treatment: Chemotherapy

"Role of Chemotherapy in Breast Cancer," Hussain SA, Palmer DH, Stevens A, et al.,
Expert Reviews in Anticancer Therapy. 2005 5(6):1095-1100.

"Side Effects of Chemotherapy and Combined Chemohormonal Therapy in Women with Early-Stage Breast Cancer," Partridge AH, Burstein HJ, *Winer EP JNCI Monographs Volume 2001, Issue 30* 135-142.

"Taxanes Alone or In Combination with Anthracyclines as First-Line Therapy of Patients with Metastatic Breast Cancer," Piccart-Gebhart MJ, Burzykowski T, Buyse M, et al., J Clin Oncol. 2008; 26(12):1980.

"Counterpoint: The Argument for Combination Chemotherapy in the Treatment of Metastatic Breast Cancer," Cianfrocca M, Gradishar WJ *Journal of the National Comprehensive Cancer Network* 2007 5 771-773

Medical Treatment: Hormone Treatment

"Weighing the Risks and Benefits of Tamoxifen Treatment for Preventing Breast Cancer," Gail MH, Constantino JP, Bryant J., et al., *Journal of National Cancer Institute 1999* vol 91 pages 1829–1846 http://www.ncbi.nlm.nih.gov/pubmed/19821307

"Aromatase Inhibitors for Treatment of Advanced Breast Cancer in Postmenopausal Women," Gibson L, Lawrence D, Dawson C, et al. *Cochrane Database Syst Rev 2009* http://www.ncbi.nlm.nih.gov/pubmed/19821307

Medical Treatment: HER2neu-Directed Therapy

"Trastuzumab—Mechanism of Action and Use in Clinical Practice" Hudis CA *New England Journal of Medicine 2007,* Vol 357, page 39.

"Efficacy and Safety of Trastuzumab as a Single Agent in First-Line Treatment of HER2-Overexpressing Metastatic Breast Cancer," Vogel CL, Cobleigh MA, Tripathy D, et al., *Journal of Clinical Oncology.* 2002; 20(3):719.

HER2 Status and Benefit from Adjuvant Trastuzumab in Breast Cancer Paik S, Kim C, Wolmark N *New England Journal of Medicine 2008,* Vol 358, page 1409.

Adjuvant Therapy

"Effect of Chemotherapy and Hormonal Therapy for Early Breast Cancer on Recurrence and Fifteen-Year Survival: An Overview of the Randomised Trials"
Lancet 2005 365 1687-1717 Available at http://www.ncbi.nlm.nih.gov/pubmed/15894097

"Population-Based Validation of the Prognostic Model ADJUVANT! For early breast cancer," Olivotto IA, Bajdick CD, Ravdin PM, et al.
Journal of Clinical Oncology 2005 23 2716-2725 http://www.ncbi.nlm.nih.gov/pubmed/15837986

Trastuzumab After Adjuvant Chemotherapy in HER2-Positive Breast Cancer.
Piccart-Gebhart MJ, Procter M, Leyland_Jones B, et al.
New England Journal of Medicine 2006 353 1659-1672. http://www.ncbi.nlm.nih.gov/pubmed/16236737

"Gene Expression and Benefit of Chemotherapy in Women with Node-Negative, Estrogen Receptor-Positive Breast Cancer," Paik S, Tang G, Shak S, et al.
Journal of Clinical Oncology 2006 24 3726-3734. 590 http://www.ncbi.nlm.nih.gov/pubmed/16720680

"Meta-Analysis of Breast Cancer Outcomes in Adjuvant Trials of Aromatase Inhibitors Versus Tamoxifen," Dowsett M, Cuzick J, Ingle J, et al.
Journal of Clinical Oncology 2010 28 509-518 http://www.ncbi.nlm.nih.gov/pubmed/19949017

Neo-Adjuvant Therapy (Preoperative Drug Treatment)

"Preoperative Chemotherapy for Breast Cancer: Miracle or Mirage?"

Hudis C, Modi S
Journal of the American Medical Association 2007 298 2665-2667 http://www.ncbi.nlm.nih.gov/pubmed/18073362

"Neoadjuvant Treatment of Postmenopausal Breast Cancer with Anastrazole, Tamoxifen or Both in Combination: the Immediate Preoperative Anastrazole, Tamoxifen or Combined with Tamoxifen (IMPACT) Multicenter Double-Blind Randomized Trial."
Smith IE, Dowsett M, Ebbs SR, et al.
Journal of Clinical Oncology 2005 23 5108-5116 http://www.ncbi.nlm.nih.gov/pubmed/5998903

BRCA1 and 2

"Inherited Breast and Ovarian Cancer," Szabo CI, King MC
Human Molecular Genetics 1995 4 (suppl 1) 1811-1817

"BRCA1 and BRCA2: Cancer Risk and Genetic Testing,"
National Cancer Institute 2009 Available online: http://www.cancer.gov/cancertopics/factsheet/Risk/BRCA

US Preventive Services Task Force (2005). "Genetic risk assessment and BRCA mutation testing for breast and ovarian cancer susceptibility: Recommendation statement." *Annals of Internal Medicine*, 2005 143(5): 355-361

Breast Cancer Risk Factors

"Effects of Tamoxifen on Benign Breast Disease in Women at High Risk for Breast Cancer," Tan-Chiu E, Wang J, Constantino JP, et al.
Journal of the National Cancer Institute 2003 95 302-307 http://www.ncbi.nlm.nih.gov/pubmed/12591986

"Evolving Concepts in the Management of Lobular Neoplasia,"
Anderson BO, Calhoun KE, Rosen EL
Journal of the National Comprehensive Cancer Network 2006 4 511-522 http://
www.ncbi.nlm.nih.gov/pubmed/16687097

"Management of Lobular Carcinoma In-Situ and Atypical Lobular
Hyperplasia of the Breast –A Review. Hussain M, Cunnick GH, *European
Journal of Surgery Oncology* 2011 37 279-289 http://www.ncbi.nlm.nih.gov/
pubmed/21306860

Ductal Carcinoma In Situ (DCIS)

"A Prognostic Index for Ductal Carcinoma in Situ of the Breast Cancer,"
1996 77 2267-2274. http://www.ncbi.nlm.nih.gov/pubmed/8635094

"Long-Term Outcomes of Invasive Ipsilateral Breast Tumor Recurrences
after Lumpectomy in NSABP B-17 and B-24 randomized clinical trials
for DCIS," Wapnir IL, Dignam JJ, Fisher B, et al.
Journal of National Cancer Institute 2011 103 478-488 http://www.ncbi.nlm.
nih.gov/pubmed/21398619

"Effect of Tamoxifen and Radiotherapy in Women with Locally Excised
Ductal Carcinoma In Situ: Long-Term Results from the UK/ANZ DCIS
Trial," Cuzick J, Sestak I, Pinder SE, et al., Lancet Oncology 2011 12 21-
29 http://www.ncbi.nlm.nih.gov/pubmed/21145284

Breast Cancer During Pregnancy

"Emerging Therapeutic Options for Breast Cancer Chemotherapy
During Pregnancy" Mir O, Berveiller P, Ropert S, et al., *Annals Oncology
2008* 19 607-613 http://www.ncbi.nlm.nih.gov/pubmed/17921242

"Pregnancy Associated Breast Cancer," *European Journal Surgical Oncology* 2009 35 215-218, http://www.ncbi.nlm.nih.gov/pubmed/18550321

"Diagnostic and Treatment Considerations When Newly Diagnosed Breast Cancer Coincides With Pregnancy: A Case Report and Review of Literature," Nye L, Hucyk TK, Gradishar WJ J Natl Compr Canc Netw 2012;10:145-148

Inflammatory Breast Cancer
"Inflammatory Breast Cancer (IBC) and Patterns of Recurrence: Understanding the Biology of a Unique Disease," Cristofanilli M, Valero V, Buzdar AU, et al.
Cancer 2007 110 1436-1444 http://www.ncbi.nlm.nih.gov/pubmed/1769455

"Locally Advanced and Inflammatory Breast Cancer," Chia S, Swain SM, Byrd DR, et al., *Journal of Clinical Oncology* 2008 26 786-790 http://www.ncbi.nlm.nih.gov/pubmed/18258987

Follow Up After Breast Cancer Treatment
"Breast Cancer Follow-Up and Management After Primary Treatment: American Society of Clinical Oncology Clinical Practice Guideline Update," Khatcheressian JL, Hurley P, Bantug E, et al., *Journal of Clinical Oncology* 2012 31 961-965

"Clinical Practice Guidelines for the Care and Treatment of Breast Cancer: Follow-up After Treatment for Breast Cancer" (summary of the 2005 update)
Grunfeld E, Dhesy-Thind S, Levine M
Canadian Medical Association Journal 2005 172 (10) 1319-1320

Male Breast Cancer

Giordano SH, Buzdar AU, Hortobagyi GN, "Breast Cancer in Men," *Annals of Internal Medicine* 2002 137 678-687 http://www.ncbi.nlm.nih.gov/pubmed/12379069

"A Review of the Diagnosis and Management of Male Breast Cancer," Giordano SH,
The Oncologist 2005 10 471-479.

About the Author

Dr. Dennis L. Citrin is a board-certified medical oncologist with more than three decades of experience. Specializing in treating advanced and complex breast cancer, Dr. Citrin works with a team of experts to help patients fight breast cancer at Cancer Treatment Centers of America.

Dr. Citrin earned his medical degree at the University of Glasgow in Scotland. He then completed a residency in internal medicine at the university. Following this, he completed three years of research in breast cancer, leading to his PhD. He was then awarded a Medical Research Council Fellowship in Cancer Medicine, which brought him to the University of Wisconsin-Madison.

After completing a fellowship in Human Oncology (cancer medicine) at the University of Wisconsin, Dr. Citrin served on the faculty of several medical schools over the next twenty years, including the University of Wisconsin, University of California in San Diego, Albert Einstein College of Medicine in Bronx, New York, and Northwestern University Medical School in Chicago, before entering private practice.

Prior to joining Cancer Treatment Centers of America in 2004, Dr. Citrin served patients in private practice and as a staff member at Northwestern Memorial Hospital in Chicago.

Dr. Citrin is a member of several professional associations, including the American Society of Clinical Oncology, the American Association for Cancer Research and the Chicago Medical Society. His research has been presented at numerous national and international conferences, and has been published extensively over the years in journals such as *Cancer* and the *Journal of Clinical Oncology*.